T0288837

Preventing, Identifying, and Treating Prescription Drug Misuse Among Active-Duty Service Members

Rosalie Liccardo Pacula, Sarah B. Hunter, Allison J. Ober,
Karen Chan Osilla, Raffaele Vardavas, Janice C. Blanchard,
David DeVries, Emmanuel F. Drabo, Kristin J. Leuschner,
Warren Stewart, Jennifer Walters

Prepared for the Office of the Secretary of Defense
Approved for public release; distribution unlimited

For more information on this publication, visit www.rand.org/t/RR1345

Library of Congress Cataloging-in-Publication Data is available for this publication.
ISBN: 978-0-8330-9667-8

Published by the RAND Corporation, Santa Monica, Calif.
© Copyright 2016 RAND Corporation
RAND® is a registered trademark.

Support RAND
Make a tax-deductible charitable contribution at
www.rand.org/giving/contribute

www.rand.org

Preface

The U.S. military is keenly interested in curtailing substance misuse among those in its ranks. However, prescription drug misuse (PDM) poses a new type of threat that might be increasing in this population. PDM, particularly of opioid analgesics, can occur among active-duty service members either because of medically indicated use from injuries for which the drug is subsequently overused or because of misuse of others' medication. The U.S. Department of Defense is seeking information on how prescription drug use and misuse among service members affects the military and what promising practices can be applied to the military context to prevent and manage (i.e., treat) PDM among military personnel. The Deputy Assistant Secretary of Defense for Readiness asked the RAND Corporation to assist it with these efforts by conducting three tasks: an extensive literature review of the current standards for preventing, identifying, and treating PDM within the military and civilian health systems; assessing, through in-person interviews with frontline medical providers, how widely those practices have been adopted in military medical facilities; and developing a tool that the military could use for projecting current and future rates of PDM among active-duty personnel. This report summarizes the findings from the literature review, documents the process and findings from qualitative interviews on this topic among military health staff, presents the framework for the tool to predict future trends in PDM, and provides key insights based on all of these tasks.

This research was sponsored by the Deputy Assistant Secretary of Defense for Readiness and conducted within the Forces and Resources

Policy Center of the RAND National Defense Research Institute, a federally funded research and development center sponsored by the Office of the Secretary of Defense, the Joint Staff, the Unified Combatant Commands, the Navy, the Marine Corps, the defense agencies, and the defense Intelligence Community.

For more information on the RAND Forces and Resources Policy Center, see www.rand.org/nsrd/ndri/centers/frp or contact the director (contact information is provided on the web page).

Contents

Figures and Tables

Figures

Tables

Summary

Analyses of medical and pharmacy claims and drug-screening data from fiscal year 2010 show that nearly one-third of active-duty service members (ADSMs) have received at least one prescription for an opioid, central nervous–system depressant, or stimulant, and well over one-quarter (26.4 percent) receive at least one prescription opioid during this period (Jeffery, May, et al., 2014). The U.S. Department of Defense (DoD) defines prescription drug misuse (PDM) as either medication misuse caused by using it too frequently or in higher doses than prescribed or medication use without a prescription (Bray, Pemberton, Hourani, et al., 2009). PDM is an increasingly common problem in both civilian and military populations. Anonymous surveys of active-duty military personnel suggest an increase of PDM (Bray, Pemberton, Lane, et al., 2010). This parallels the recent trend of PDM seen in the civilian population, in which there is growing concern among policymakers, the Centers for Disease Control and Prevention, and other stakeholders about nonmedical initiation and use of pain relievers (Substance Abuse and Mental Health Services Administration [SAMHSA], 2011).

The misuse of prescribed substances is of special concern for the military because of its potential impact on military readiness, the health and well-being of military personnel, and associated health care costs. However, addressing this problem poses special challenges in the detection and prevention of misuse because of the important clinical indications for which these drugs might be prescribed. Effective strategies are needed to reduce the risk of PDM and ensure safe use.

To help DoD address these issues, the RAND National Defense Research Institute conducted three related efforts that could provide useful information for assisting the military in preventing, identifying, and treating PDM: a review of guidelines and empirical literature for the prevention, identification, and treatment of PDM in clinical settings (both military and civilian) to help identify best practices; the development of an analytic tool that can be used to predict trends and changes in PDM among ADSMs today and into the future; and interviews with civilian and military providers at military installations. This report includes information gleaned from each of these three major activities and summarizes common themes from across them. Of course, as is true with any study, to some degree the limitations of the approaches taken, which we describe in detail in each of the chapters, shape the findings and insights, which should be viewed within the contexts of the strengths and limitations of the study.

Evidence-Based Practices for Preventing, Identifying, and Treating Prescription Drug Misuse

We reviewed all publicly available DoD policies and clinical guidelines and examined the empirical literature to identify practices for preventing, identifying, and treating PDM. We were specifically interested in identifying evidence-based practices for PDM (rather than substance abuse more broadly) and understanding whether they have been tested and were being used in military settings. Our project officer defined prescription drugs of interest based on DoD interest (see Table S.1) and included opioids (i.e., morphine, codeine, hydrocodone, oxycodone, methadone, fentanyl, and meperidine), stimulants (i.e., methylphenidate and a combination of dextroamphetamine and amphetamine), benzodiazepines, and barbiturates.

U.S. Department of Defense Directives Provide Little Guidance on Preventing and Managing Prescription Drug Misuse

The 20 DoD directives we reviewed provide little guidance specifically pertaining to the management of prescription drug use and misuse

Table S.1
Prescription Drugs of Interest for Our Study

Class	Generic	Common Brand Names
Opioids	Morphine	Duramorph, DepoDur, Astramorph, Infumorph
	Codeine	
	Hydrocodone	Zohydro Extended Release, Hysingla Extended Release
	Oxycodone	Oxycontin, Roxicodone, Oxecta
	Methadone	Methadose, Diskets, Dolophine
	Fentanyl	Duragesic, Abstral, Subsys, Ionsys, Sublimaze
	Meperidine	Demerol
Stimulants	Methylphenidate	Ritalin, Daytrana, Concerta, Methylin, Aptensio
	Dextroamphetamine with amphetamine	Adderall
Benzodiazepines		
Barbiturates		

within the military. Instead, many focus on defining PDM and the consequences following identification, such as the process for adjudicating urine tests. Some directives included so-called limited-use policies that were inconsistently presented alongside zero tolerance guidelines. The majority of the clinical guidelines reviewed (both military-specific and others) focus on prescription opioids, with little guidance on the management of misuse of other classes of prescription drugs. Current DoD clinical recommendations for prescription opioid misuse appear to be similar to non-DoD clinical guidelines. Most guidelines note the lack of strong research evidence for many of the current care recommendations that address the prevention of misuse of prescription opioids.

All guidelines, both military and civilian, support an initial assessment to evaluate risk of PDM at the time a provider is considering prescribing the opioid. Guidelines provide consistent support for conducting a comprehensive assessment of a patient's medical history, including history of substance abuse and comorbid psychiatric and medical history, before initiating therapy (Cantrill et al., 2012; Chou, Fanciullo, et al., 2009; Manchikanti et al., 2012a, 2012b; Thorson et al., 2013). However, there is little supporting evidence concerning the effectiveness of approaches, such as screening exams, to predict patient characteristics for misuse. Many guidelines recommend written management plans and urine drug screens when there is a high risk of PDM despite limited evidence of these tools' effectiveness (Cantrill et al., 2012; Chou, Fanciullo, et al., 2009; Manchikanti et al., 2012a, 2012b; Thorson et al., 2013).

The current DoD guidelines regarding substance use discuss general approaches to treatment and are generally not focused on specific management of PDM (Management of Substance Use Disorders Work Group, 2009). The problem of opioid abuse is particularly challenging, given the need to balance the benefits of pain management and the risk of addiction (Prescription Drug Abuse Subcommittee, 2013). There is also a paucity of studies addressing the specific problem of prescription opioid abuse in the broader literature, and few empirical studies specifically address the prevention or treatment of PDM.

In 2009, then–U.S. Army Surgeon General LTG Eric B. Schoomaker led a multidisciplinary task force to address pain management issues in the military (Office of the Army Surgeon General, 2010). This task force stressed the importance of deemphasizing opioid therapy for the management of chronic pain and having providers focus more on problems of prescription opioid abuse. However, as this systematic review shows, more evidence is needed to help guide proper implementation of task-force recommendations with respect to alternatives to writing prescriptions.

Given the complexities of managing patients suffering with chronic, as well as acute, pain; the tremendous potential for these patients in particular to misuse prescription drugs, as well as other substances (McLellan and Turner, 2010; Nuckols et al., 2014); and the fact that providers typically lack general knowledge or training on how to deal with these patients, it would seem that, alongside remedial training of existing health care providers, immediate training of all new military health care providers would be useful. In particular, this training would allow the military the opportunity to promote and adopt a single standardized assessment tool for identifying a variety of substances that might be misused (e.g., prescription opioid, alcohol, benzodiazepines); train providers on how to use the tool and what to do when someone is identified as being at risk; provide clear directives on the military's position regarding pharmacotherapy's role in treating opioid misuse (or alcohol dependence); and provide clarity on policies, protocols, and clinical guidelines to follow for these particularly difficult and unique cases.

Analytic Tool to Predict Trends and Changes in Prescription Drug Misuse Among Active-Duty Service Members

To know when to intervene with those experiencing PDM problems, one must first know where these people might be identified. To assist the military in its effort to better understand the extent to which PDM stems from medically indicated use (i.e., misuse that stems from a having a prescription for a highly addictive prescription) and non-medical use (i.e., misuse of a prescription drug that was not prescribed to that person), we developed an analytic tool that, once populated with data that the military owns, can serve as a valuable means for understanding the dynamics of the current PDM problem. In addition to identifying for policymakers the share of PDM that emerges from medically indicated use versus nonmedical use and how these will change over time, the analytic tool can be used to identify nodes in the model at which prevention and treatment resources might more effectively be concentrated so as to more efficiently and effectively tackle the problem. Prevention and treatment dollars are limited, so understanding the key factors (nodes, in our model) that drive higher rates of misuse will also tell decisionmakers where limited resources might be focused so as to more efficiently reduce the problem.

In addition to providing military officials with a better understanding of the incidence and prevalence of PDM beyond what can be determined from regular drug testing and occasional survey data, the analytic tool can be used to forecast how the incidence and prevalence of PDM will change in the future if current practices stay the course. For example, the analytic tool can be used to project how PDM might grow among those with medical indications vis-à-vis growth in the non–medical use population. Alternatively, the analytic tool could be used to project how current trajectories might change with a change in any of the tool's underlying assumptions, such as the rate of heavy use among the medically indicated, escalation rates from light to heavy use, the rate at which people enter treatment, and the relative effectiveness of different treatments. Using the tool in this manner is commonly referred to as *predictive forecasting*. Alternatively, the analytic tool could be restructured to accommodate different classes of prescription drugs individually (e.g., narcotics only, stimulants only) and then could be used to describe patterns of use and trends for particular prescription drug trajectories.

Like the value of any epidemiological model of health behavior, the value of the tool we propose here will depend on the reliability of estimates obtained for the various assumptions that make up the model that underlies it. Our scan of the data fields contained in TRI-CARE (the military health care system that includes insurance claims), the DoD Health Related Behaviors Survey and drug-testing data suggest that sufficient data exist to develop empirically driven assumptions for the model variables needed. Standard techniques for checking reliability and validity of the model would be necessary, but, assuming that the model is shown to be both externally valid and reliable, the tool proposed here could provide military health leaders with guidance on how to target limited prevention and treatment dollars toward the key factors that appear to drive higher rates of misuse.

Qualitative Interviews

Finally, we conducted semistructured interviews with military personnel to better understand perceptions of the nature and extent of PDM among ADSMs; current practices and policies to prevent, identify, and treat PDM; and barriers to effective management of PDM. To collect information from personnel with relevant experience, we developed a strategic sampling of military bases with medical treatment facilities (MTFs) in regions of the conterminous United States where selective prescription drugs, particularly opiates and benzodiazepines, were frequently administered in 2010, according to evidence in the TRICARE pharmacy claim data. TRICARE is a health care insurance program of the U.S. Military Health System (MHS) (formerly known as the Civilian Health and Medical Program for the Uniformed Services) that covers care not available through U.S. military medical service or public health service facilities. Our goal was to include bases from each of the service branches, although our ability to reach base commanders and obtain necessary approvals for the interviews within the time frame allotted for the study greatly influenced the list of final bases we included in our sample. Our final sample included 66 health providers at nine MTFs across the services.

In general, providers reported that PDM is a problem among ADSMs and that PDM most commonly occurs among those who, at one time, had medically indicated use. Although diversion of prescription drugs for nonmedical purposes occurs, most providers we interviewed do not think the prevalence of this type of misuse is high. The providers we interviewed perceive that PDM occurs because of a combination of factors, including the high prevalence of pain among ADSMs; psychological vulnerability to addiction; and provider problems, such as overprescribing and lack of training and expertise in recognizing PDM and in treating people who have chronic pain.

Although the providers we interviewed had some knowledge of clinical practice guidelines for chronic pain, as well as DoD directives around substance abuse and PDM, practices and adherence tend to vary by provider and MTF in those we accessed, with providers noting the need for more-consistent guidelines and greater adherence. For example, most of the MTFs reported using so-called sole-provider agreements, which are agreements between health care providers and patients that limit patients to a single prescribing physician for all medications (i.e., a sole-provider agreement) and might have other requirements regarding refills, frequency of medical appointments, and consequences of misuse (a high-risk medication agreement). However, even clinics within the same MTFs have different patient criteria for utilizing agreements, the terms of the agreements, and the names of the agreements. Additionally, despite policies that state otherwise, providers perceive that typically a zero tolerance policy around PDM parallels the policy for illicit-drug use. However, they also reported that decisions around PDM are made on a case-by-case basis. This discrepancy seems to lead to uncertainty about how to handle PDM. The providers with whom we spoke mentioned that they would like to see more-consistent guidelines, more-consistent monitoring of and adherence to clinical practice guidelines, and more guidance around administrative outcomes for ADSMs with PDM.

Evidence-based practices, such as standardized assessments for potential misuse and behavioral and pharmacological treatments, are not typically implemented in primary care or emergency room settings, according to our sample. Some pain specialists employ screening procedures, and there have been some efforts to bring screening to primary care and family practice settings, but with little success. Although providers acknowledge that there is very little time to conduct assessments, as well as a lack of understanding about what to do if a patient with pain is susceptible to PDM (according to an assessment), they see the value of having a more standardized tool for assessing the potential for PDM. Use of medication-assisted treatment for PDM was not mentioned. However, when prompted, some providers noted that medication-assisted treatment might present a challenge for providers: To prescribe Suboxone (a medication for opioid dependence containing buprenorphine and naloxone) to treat addiction, a provider must have a special U.S. Drug Enforcement Administration license. Providers with whom we spoke also lack understanding about their role in treating opioid dependence pharmacologically within the MTF. Naltrexone, both injectable and oral, is a viable option for treating some opioid-dependent patients (SAMHSA, 2015), but the providers with whom we spoke are not familiar with the medication, not comfortable providing medication for opioid dependence, or not aware of the regulations around doing so.

The greatest challenge in managing PDM facing the providers with whom we spoke is the lack of a clear definition of PDM, therefore leading to challenges in appropriately preventing, identifying, and treating PDM. Also, a lack of clarity around the policies, protocols, and guidelines across MTFs and bases leads to inconsistent practices. Providers offered a variety of recommendations for addressing these challenges, including expanding resources for preventing, identifying, and treating PDM by embedding case managers and clinical pharmacists into clinics; having pain specialists at each clinic; offering patient-centered practices, such as complementary approaches to medication; improving patient education around prescriptions, including the provision of self-management tools; clarifying and supporting adherence to guidelines and policies; improving electronic systems to enhance tracking of all prescriptions; and increasing provider training and interdisciplinary support and coordination of care.

Additionally, the substance abuse treatment providers with whom we spoke reported that there might be a lack of capacity to treat PDM on base as opposed to at a nonmilitary treatment center. Some providers said that MTF substance abuse treatment programs typically treat only alcohol problems, while others reported also treating PDM but not having specific tools for doing so. Some providers reported using educational treatment models and others reported including members with PDM into treatment groups with other illicit-drug users. The substance abuse providers with whom we spoke would like to see more-tailored educational and treatment protocols for ADSMs with PDM.

Key Insights from This Work and Strategies for Going Forward

Determining what should be done about PDM is a complex task. As indicated in our systematic literature review, few available evidence-based solutions focus specifically on the prevention, identification, or treatment of PDM in the military or civilian practice. Moreover, the DoD regulations are complex, emphasizing a general zero tolerance approach to drugs with little mention of addressing prescription drug use and misuse. Furthermore, the providers we interviewed made many recommendations with limited knowledge of the significant barriers to implementing the change suggested (e.g., distributing standardized guidelines on identification and treatment of PDM requires existence of effective evidence-based models). However, given the information gleaned from our literature review and interviews with selected providers, we can offer the following insights for consideration and potential paths forward.

Implement and Parameterize the Compartmental Model Developed in This Report to Enable a Clear Assessment of the Extent to Which the Current Prescription Drug Misuse Problem Within the Military Stems from Abuse Following Legitimate Medical Need or Simple Inappropriate Use

Military leadership can use the model, once parameterized and tested, to track the evolution of the PDM problem over time (based on trends in key characteristics driving the problem over time) and identify the extent to which particular policy approaches (e.g., harsh penalties targeting misusers, or broader implementation of step-down therapies and pain management techniques for patients suffering from severe injuries causing pain) might be effective at addressing the unique PDM problem that the military faces.

Dedicate Resources to Providing Remedial Training and Support to All Military Health Care Providers in the Identification and Treatment of Substance Abuse in Patients

Our findings provide justification for clinical training of all new and existing medical personnel on identifying and treating addictions (i.e., a comprehensive course providing information on identifying early signs of all addictive behaviors, not just those most problematic today). In doing so, the military can address the current PDM problem and educate its providers on how to identify future potential health problems, such as problems with benzodiazepines, alcohol, or even e-cigarettes. However, the military needs to do more than just provide training. In particular, it needs to make sure that the training that is provided is indeed scientifically supported and effective. It must make sure that the training is easy for providers to access and use, even when time is limited with patients. Remedial courses with military health care providers before they are assigned to their posts is one way to engage providers early on and educate them on preferred practices, such as the use of a single standardized, evidence-based screening tool for identification of substance misuse across the MHS and what to do if someone screens positive using that tool.

The military needs to go further than just providing training to providers, however, for the training to be truly effective. The military needs to be aware of and address for providers the system- and patient-level barriers that make providing linked care so difficult. It could remove patient barriers through the broad-scale implementation of a modified limited-use policy, such as the Army's Confidential Alcohol Treatment and Education Program (CATEP), but applied to PDM. Health system barriers might be overcome through electronic connectivity between providers, brief case-management strategies, and supportive care activities to better connect care received in the medical and specialty treatment settings (Cucciare and Timko, 2015; Molfenter et al., 2012; Rapp et al., 2008). These are just a couple of strategies currently being adopted within the civilian health care system in light of mandates associated with the Patient Protection and Affordable Care Act (Pub. L. 111-148, 2010) to better integrate behavioral and medical health care for people suffering from substance use disorders (Humphreys and Frank, 2014; Ghitza and Tai, 2014).

Facilitate Interdisciplinary Provider Coordination in Approaches to Identifying and Treating Prescription Drug Misuse, as Well as the Transition to Integrated Care

Although effective coordination of care through electronic medical records might be years away, changes in civilian and military health care systems that include care coordination through patient-centered medical homes (PCMHs) provide a natural opportunity for expanded prevention, identification, and treatment of PDM. Several models of PCMHs are currently being evaluated within the military sector (Nathan, 2013). In MTFs that have already begun to make these changes, providers reported greater collaboration between providers since the institution of PCMHs through the use of embedded case managers and behavioral health therapists to facilitate chart reviews and communication about and management of ADSMs with PDM and at risk for PDM. Given that service integration is relatively new, it is important to continue to monitor these efforts to help inform how to best design these systems for the future.

For Those Suffering with Chronic Pain, Expand the Availability of and Access to Pain Management and Patient-Centered Practices Within the Military Health System

It was clear from our discussion with providers that pain management and patient-centered, complementary services are not readily available or accessible to those suffering from chronic pain. Providers believe that these practices can support treatment for patients with chronic pain, but there are few within the MHS who provide these services and, where they are available, waiting lists can be long. Treatment outside of the MHS is also possible, but coverage for that care might be limited, and the tracking of these alternative treatments is often difficult.

Given the unique challenges of managing PDM patients suffering from either acute or chronic pain, as well as the lack of general medical training on how to treat these patients, the military could benefit from the development of some remedial training for all new military health care providers on this topic as well. This training, which could commence before the medical and paramedical personnel are first assigned to their posts, would provide the military the opportunity to educate its medical providers on how to use a single standardized assessment tool for identifying pain patients who are at risk of substance abuse (e.g., PDM or alcohol) and what to do when ADSMs are identified as at risk from these assessments. Remedial training for existing medical personnel encountering these types of patients should also be encouraged. Clear directives could be provided to all medical and paramedical personnel on the policies, protocols, and clinical guidelines that the military believes are the most effective to follow for these patients, as well as provide clear directives to providers regarding the role of pharmacotherapies for treating opioid (or even alcohol) misuse.

Encourage the Use of State Prescription Drug Monitoring Programs

Existing state prescription drug monitoring programs (PDMPs) are infrequently used and fraught with barriers for those providing medical services within the military. Enhanced policies and procedures to direct military providers to PDMPs to check for purchases made outside the TRICARE system would help reduce risk of overprescribing and overcome some, although not all, of the barriers. Potential challenges to this approach include making sure that someone at each military medical facility or clinic has access to the state's PDMP (different states have different rules regarding who is allowed to access their PDMPs). Potential policy changes might be needed to fully realize the benefit, such as allowing military health providers access to state PDMPs or requiring prescriptions purchased through TRICARE to be included in state PDMPs. However, these policy changes are likely to happen far more expeditiously than the adoption of a military-wide PDMP that also has access to state PDMPs, which is likely to be the only way for any PDMP to reduce prescription drug abuse among active service members and their dependents, but considerably more costly to build and implement.

Determine Whether Military Substance Abuse Programs Should Provide Unique, Prescription Drug Misuse–Focused Treatment for Service Members Who Develop Dependence on Prescription Medications

The military should explore the potential use of pharmacological maintenance, tapering, and anticraving medications for opiate dependence (e.g., buprenorphine/naloxone or oral, injectable, or extended-release naltrexone). These treatments have been shown to be potentially effective for opioid-dependent populations (SAMHSA, 2015). Although there are administrative and practical complexities to providing some of these pharmacological treatments for substance dependence to ADSMs, adoption of these forms of treatment could facilitate and expedite recovery and reintegration of service members into active duty. Other evidence-based behavioral therapies tailored for people misusing prescription drugs, including those suffering from opioid misuse and xxii Preventing, Identifying, and Treating Prescription Drug Misuse

chronic pain, also exist (e.g., Rawson, Shoptaw, et al., 1995; Rawson, Marinelli-Casey, et al., 2004).

If the number of ADSMs who experience PDM is expected to grow in the future, which the full implementation of our proposed analytic tool could reveal, then attention to building and sustaining the internal treatment capacity for PDM will definitely be needed. Although it is expensive to seek broader-scale adoption of any of the treatment approaches described in the previous paragraph, the cost-effectiveness of doing so would dramatically decrease if the size of the hidden population is substantially larger than the relatively small number of ADSMs who seek or receive treatment within the military today. Thus, use of a forecasting tool, such as the one we describe in this report, could be very helpful for evaluating the desirability of pursuing the development of any particular approach broad scale at military treatment centers.

Consider Adoption, Implementation, and Improved Dissemination of a U.S. Department of Defense–Wide Limited-Use Policy

DoD policies toward substance abuse are quite complex but generally emphasize a zero tolerance approach to controlled substance use, including the nonmedical use of a prescription drug. However, some of the services have adopted what is commonly referred to as limited-use policies, in which people who misuse prescription drugs can, under very specific conditions, self-refer to treatment and avoid harsh disciplinary actions or administrative separation. These programs are modeled on the successful Army CATEP, which was implemented with the explicit purpose of encouraging ADSMs to self-refer to treatment for alcohol problems before a reportable event occurs. Limited-use policies exist today in the Army (Army Regulation 600-85, 2012 [Headquarters, Department of the Army, 2012b], p. 25, § 4-2) and Navy (Chief of Naval Operations Instruction 5350.4D, 2009 [Director, Personal Readiness and Community Support Branch, 2009], enc. 2, § e, p. 12) for those suffering from PDM, although they vary in terms of allowable behaviors and remain quite complex to fully interpret in light of the harsh zero tolerance language that surrounds them. Very few military medical providers with whom we spoke made any mention of the ability to self-refer to treatment, even though these policies exist, and those who did retained their belief that the risk of administrative separation from the military was a strong deterrent. Thus, either (1) broad awareness of these policies has not been achieved or (2) they do not represent a true change in the previous culture or perception of PDM as an illegal behavior worthy of separation from the military. Our reading of these policies suggests that expanding PDM limited-use policies to more service branches might be possible, making PDM function more like alcohol use does in CATEP. However, legal experts more familiar with the specific nuances of these policies and legal precedent within each of the service branches would need to be consulted before such a conclusion could be definitively made.

Of course, the insights from this study need to be considered in light of the study's limitations. In particular, there was limited evidence of effective strategies at the time in which we conducted our systematic review of the literature, but substantial attention given to the problem of PDM in the civilian sector in the past year might have generated some new evidence. Additional limitations of our study include the use of a limited sample of military medical providers and MTFs and missing data to inform the mathematical model. Before considering action on any of the study's key insights, it might be wise to conduct a more comprehensive survey of military health providers to obtain a more representative perspective of providers' barriers, challenges, and recommendations of providers, one that can consider differences that are likely to exist across regions, military facilities, and provider types.

Acknowledgments

We would like to acknowledge the tremendous support and assistance that CAPT Kevin L. Klette and LTC Thomas Martin provided to the team. Walid F. Gellad provided guidance regarding proper identification of opioids and benzodiazepines in the TRICARE claim data, and Mark Totten provided analytic support and summary information that we used to identify regions for interviews. Finally, we would like to acknowledge the additional guidance and support from our colleagues within the RAND National Defense Research Institute, particularly John D. Winkler, Kristie L. Gore, and Sarah O. Meadows, in addition to three reviewers who provided us with excellent comments that greatly improved the quality of this report: Charles C. Engel, James Broyles, and Charles O'Brien.

Abbreviations

ADAPT	Alcohol and Drug Abuse Prevention and Treatment
ADSM	active-duty service member
AFI	Air Force instruction
AHLTA	Armed Forces Health Longitudinal Technology Application
AR	Army regulation
ASAP	Army Substance Abuse Program
BUMEDINST	Bureau of Medicine and Surgery instruction
CATEP	Confidential Alcohol Treatment and Education Program
CHCS	Composite Health Care System
CHUP	chronic pain, high utilizer, polypharmacy
COMM	Current Opioid Misuse Measure
CPG	clinical practice guideline
DEA	U.S. Drug Enforcement Administration
DoD	U.S. Department of Defense
DoDD	Department of Defense directive

DoDI	Department of Defense instruction
ECHO	Extension for Community Healthcare Outcomes
EMR	electronic medical record
ER	emergency room
HRBS	Health Related Behaviors Survey
IOM	Institute of Medicine
MEDCOM	U.S. Army Medical Command
MHS	Military Health System
MPDATP	Military Personnel Drug Abuse Testing Program
MTF	medical treatment facility
NP	nurse practitioner
OASD	Office of the Assistant Secretary of Defense
OPNAVINST	Chief of Naval Operations instruction
PA	physician assistant
PCM	primary care manager
PCMH	patient-centered medical home
PCP	primary care physician
PDM	prescription drug misuse
PDMP	prescription drug monitoring program
POC	point of contact
SAMHSA	Substance Abuse and Mental Health Services Administration
SARP	Substance Abuse Rehabilitation Program

SOAPP-R	Screener and Opioid Assessment for Patients with Pain—Revised
SP	sole provider
SUD	substance use disorder
UA	urinalysis
VA	U.S. Department of Veterans Affairs
VTC	video teleconference
WTU	Warrior Transition Unit

CHAPTER ONE

Introduction

Prescription drug misuse (PDM), particularly misuse of opioid analgesics, is an increasingly common problem in both military and civilian populations. The term *misuse* includes a range of problematic uses, from simply taking a medication more frequently or in greater amounts than prescribed to taking a medication in order to attain a "high" (Bray, Pemberton, Hourani, et al., 2009). In the military, medical providers distribute pain relievers both domestically and internationally for management of service members' pain; however, these drugs can lead to abuse, addiction, and other problems, particularly among service members suffering with comorbid mental health problems (Seal et al., 2012). Analyses of medical and pharmacy claims and drug-screening data from fiscal year 2010 show that nearly one-third of active-duty service members (ADSMs) have received at least one prescription for an opioid, central nervous–system depressant, or stimulant (Jeffery, May, et al., 2014) and that well over one-quarter (26.4 percent) receive at least one prescription for opioids during the 12-month fiscal year (Jeffery, May, et al., 2014).

These rates suggest the need to address potential misuse among active-duty personnel. Moreover, the burgeoning black market for these types of drugs can make them more available to all consumers, including service members. The same analysis examining medical prescriptions for opioids among ADSMs showed that just under 1 percent (0.7 percent) of the total force received more than a 90-day prescription for opioids, which is just one of several measures that is frequently used to identify inappropriate medical use of prescription opioids (Cochran et al., 2015).

The misuse of prescribed substances is a concern for the military because of its potential impact on military readiness, the health and well-being of military personnel, and associated health care costs (Jeffery, May, et al., 2014). For example, PDM is associated with such negative consequences as drug dependence, drug overdose, suicides, and accidents (Bohnert, Roeder, and Ilgen, 2010; Golub and Bennett, 2013; Wu et al., 2010). A recent report by the Army indicates that this is a growing problem; among active-duty Army personnel, drug-overdose deaths more than doubled between 2006 and 2011, and 68 percent of these deaths involved prescription medications (Headquarters, Department of the Army, 2012a).

The military has historically been actively engaged in curtailing substance misuse among those in its ranks. Memorandum 62884, which Deputy Secretary of Defense Frank C. Carlucci issued in December 1981, authorized the initiation of punitive actions, including courts martial or administrative separation for drug use. Prior to 1981, random drug testing existed but with the primary purpose of identifying service members who were using and needed to be transferred to treatment. The policy change was not viewed as a deterrent. In May 1981, a major aircraft accident on board the USS *Nimitz* cost an estimated $150 million; drugs were identified as a contributing factor to the accident, and it was because of this that Carlucci issued memorandum 62884.

PDM poses a new type of threat, however, and drug testing might not be as useful a strategy for deterring use as it has been for other substances of abuse because of the difficulty in assessing clinically appropriate medical use of these potentially addictive drugs, particularly in managing pain associated with physical injuries. Determining exactly when a patient with a medical prescription crosses the line of appropriate use into PDM can be very difficult. For simplicity, throughout this report, we refer to someone who has a medical need for a prescription drug as a *medically indicated user* and that person's use simply as *medically indicated use*; we refer to someone who is not using under medical supervision as a *nonmedical user* and that person's use as *nonmedical use*.

This problem is not unique to the military. However, the Military Health System (MHS) is particularly well situated to develop metrics for identifying the problem because of its comprehensive and integrative prescription and medical care administrative data, which TRICARE maintains. TRICARE is the MHS health care insurance program and was formerly known as the Civilian Health and Medical Program for the Uniformed Services. Moreover, it has even greater incentives to prevent and treat the problem in light of the kind of work service members do and the presumed impact that PDM has on readiness.

Effective strategies are needed to reduce the risk of PDM and to ensure safe use of necessary medication. To assist the U.S. Department of Defense (DoD) with its efforts, researchers from the RAND National Defense Research Institute used three different research strategies in this project to assist the military in preventing, identifying, and treating PDM. First, we conducted a systematic review of evidence-based practices for the prevention and treatment of PDM, examining relevant DoD-issued policies and directives, and reviewed the clinical practice guidelines (CPGs) for identifying, preventing, and treating PDM in both the military and civilian sectors. Second, we constructed an analytic tool that, once populated with data not available to us, the military can use to estimate the current number of ADSMs engaging in PDM and predict trends based on population demographics and anticipated injury rates. Third, we conducted qualitative interviews with a sample of medical providers at nine military treatment facilities to obtain information on their perceptions of the PDM problem, their knowledge of current directives and clinical guidelines, and their opinions of and recommendations for improving the identification and treatment of PDM among ADSMs. We performed each of these activities to provide us with better insights on how to improve current military efforts to prevent, identify, and treat PDM among ADSMs. In the following chapters, we describe each of these efforts and, in the final chapter, provide key insights from this work.

CHAPTER TWO

Literature Review of Military and Civilian Practices and Guidelines for Prescription Drug Misuse

In this chapter, we describe a comprehensive literature review that we conducted to help inform the military about the current evidence base for identifying and treating PDM (see Blanchard et al., 2016). The goal of this review was to identify evidence-based practices for the prevention, identification, and treatment of PDM, specifically to help inform future DoD efforts. The reason for the narrow focus was the prior recent release of the Institute of Medicine (IOM) review of substance abuse disorders in the military, which included sections pertaining to guidelines and policies for treating substance use more broadly (IOM, 2012). We examined current clinical guidelines and conducted a systematic review of the recent research literature to identify effective approaches for the prevention and treatment of PDM. We then compared what we learned from that with DoD policies and clinical guidelines to inform our work.

U.S. Department of Defense Policies

Our process for the review was to first identify relevant DoD policies, so that we could identify the current military strategies and clinical guidelines. We examined policies that were cited in a recent IOM report (IOM, 2012) regarding substance use in the U.S. armed forces (see Table 2.1) and identified additional policies that had been updated since that report. In these searches, we identified and reviewed 20 DoD policies. We found that these policies provide little guidance specifically pertaining to the management of prescription drug

Table 2.1
U.S. Department of Defense Policy and Directives That We Reviewed

Number	Title	Citation
DoDD 1010.1	*Military Personnel Drug Abuse Testing Program*	Assistant Secretary of Defense for Special Operations and Low-Intensity Conflict, 1999a
DoDI 1010.01	*Military Personnel Drug Abuse Testing Program (MPDATP)*	Under Secretary of Defense for Personnel and Readiness, 2012b
DoDD 1010.4	*Drug and Alcohol Abuse by DoD Personnel*	Assistant Secretary of Defense for Special Operations and Low-Intensity Conflict, 1997
DoDD 1010.4	*Drug and Alcohol Abuse by DoD Personnel*	Assistant Secretary of Defense for Special Operations and Low-Intensity Conflict, 1999b
DoDI 1010.04	*Problematic Substance Use by DoD Personnel*	Under Secretary of Defense for Personnel and Readiness, 2014
DoDI 1010.6	*Rehabilitation and Referral Services for Alcohol and Drug Abusers*	Assistant Secretary of Defense for Health Affairs, 1985
DoDI 1010.09	*DoD Civilian Employee Drug-Free Workplace Program*	Under Secretary of Defense for Personnel and Readiness, 2012a
DoDI 6490.03	*Deployment Health*	Under Secretary of Defense for Personnel and Readiness, 2011b
DoDI 6490.08	*Command Notification Requirements to Dispel Stigma in Providing Mental Health Care to Service Members*	Under Secretary of Defense for Personnel and Readiness, 2011a
Secretary of the Navy Instruction 5300.28E	*Military Substance Abuse Prevention and Control*	Assistant Secretary of the Navy for Manpower and Reserve Affairs, 2011
OPNAVINST 5350.4D	*Navy Alcohol and Drug Abuse Prevention and Control*	Director, Personal Readiness and Community Support, 2009
BUMEDINST 5350.5	*Headquarters, Bureau of Medicine and Surgery Alcohol and Drug Prevention Program*	Chief of Staff, Bureau of Medicine and Surgery, 2011

Table 2.1—Continued

Number	Title	Citation
BUMEDINST 5353.4A	*Standards for Provision of Substance Related Disorder Treatment Services*	Assistant Chief of Staff for Health Care Operations, 1999
AR 600-86	*The Army Substance Abuse Program*	Secretary of the Army, 2009
MEDCOM Regulation 40-51	*Medical Review Officers and Review of Positive Urinalysis Drug Testing Results*	Assistant Chief of Staff for Health Policy and Services, 2011
All Army Activities 062/2011	"ALARACT Changes to Length of Authorized Duration of Controlled Substance Prescriptions in MEDCOM Regulation 40-51"	Office of the Army Surgeon General, 2011
Navy Marine Corps 2931	*Drug and Alcohol Abuse Prevention and Treatment Programs*	U.S. Marine Corps, undated
Marine Corps Order 5300.17	*Marine Corps Substance Abuse Program*	Deputy Commandant for Manpower and Reserve Affairs, 2011
AFI 44-121	*Alcohol and Drug Abuse Prevention and Treatment (ADAPT) Program*	Deputy Surgeon General of the Air Force, 2011
AFI 44-172 Air Force Guidance Memorandum 1	*Guidance Memorandum to Air Force Instruction (AFI) 44-172, Mental Health*	Air Force Surgeon General, 2012

NOTE: DoDD = DoD directive. DoDI = DoD instruction. BUMEDINST = Bureau of Medicine and Surgery instruction. AR = Army regulation. MEDCOM = U.S. Army Medical Command. AFI = Air Force instruction.

use and misuse. Instead, many focus on drug abuse more generally, defining the PDM problem and the consequences following identification, such as the process for adjudicating urine tests. Moreover, the guidelines generally emphasized a zero tolerance approach toward drug abuse with few mentioning limited-use policies. For example, Chief of Naval Operations Instruction (OPNAVINST) 5350.4D, *Navy Alcohol and Drug Abuse Prevention and Control* (Director, Personal Readiness and Community Support Branch, 2009), provides an overarching statement that the Navy's policy toward drug abuse is zero tolerance, as indicated in the first sentence of the drug testing program overview and several other times throughout. The policy defines drug abuse as the wrongful or unintended use of controlled substances. However, the instruction also provides some limited-use scenarios, such as,

> if a commanding officer determines [that] a positive drug test reported by a DoD drug-screening laboratory was not wrongful use (e.g., prescribed medicine), commands must notify [the director of the Personal Readiness and Community Support Branch] via official correspondence, explaining the circumstances that warranted such determination.

It also specifies an option for self-referral: "members who self-refer as a result of prescription medication may be retained on active duty, provided [that] commands submit a request to [the director of the Personal Readiness and Community Support Branch] that explains why the positive urinalysis is not a drug abuse incident." In sum, the policies reviewed were complex, making them challenging to follow and potentially sending mixed messages.

Clinical Practice Guidelines, Consensus Statements, and Published Systematic Reviews

Next, we reviewed current clinical guidelines, consensus statements, and published systematic reviews that were completed in 2014. We used the Agency for Healthcare Research and Quality's National Guideline Clearinghouse to identify CPGs. The clearinghouse is an online searchable database of guidelines from a variety of organizations compiled from systematic reviews of the literature (Agency for Healthcare Research and Quality, undated). The team also performed an online search of well-known organizations that publish clinical resources for PDM, specifically focusing on identifying guidelines that national U.S. organizations have issued. From these practice guidelines, we examined references to published systematic reviews and pulled them for further background review.

In sum, we examined six CPGs, five consensus documents, and seven published systematic reviews. Two of the CPGs were military specific: *VA/DoD Clinical Practice Guideline for Management of Substance Use Disorders* (Management of Substance Use Disorders Work Group, 2009) and *VA/DoD Clinical Practice Guideline for the Management of Opioid Therapy for Chronic Pain* (Management of Opioid Therapy for Chronic Pain Working Group, 2010). The majority of the military clinical guidelines reviewed focused on prescription opioids, with little guidance on the management of misuse of other classes of prescription drugs. Current DoD clinical recommendations for opioid prescription misuse are joint with the U.S. Department of Veterans Affairs (VA), not unlike those for other areas of substance abuse, and appear to be similar to non-DoD clinical guidelines.

Most guidelines note the lack of strong research evidence for many of the current care recommendations that address the prevention of misuse of prescription opioids. For example, all CPGs we identified, both military and civilian, support an initial assessment to evaluate risk of PDM at the time a provider is considering prescribing an opioid (Cantrill et al., 2012; Chou, Fanciullo, et al., 2009; Manchikanti et al., 2012a, 2012b; Thorson et al., 2013). However, there was little supporting evidence concerning the effectiveness of this approach in predicting misuse. Moreover, many guidelines recommend written management plans and urine drug screens when there is a high risk of PDM despite limited proof of these tools' effectiveness (Cantrill et al., 2012; Chou, Fanciullo, et al., 2009; Manchikanti et al., 2012a, 2012b; Thorson et al., 2013). There was also no strong evidence for the utility of chronic opioid-management plans in curbing misuse (Chou, Fanciullo, et al., 2009; Manchikanti et al., 2012a, 2012b; Thorson et al., 2013). Some guidelines recommend the use of prescription drug monitoring programs (PDMPs) to help assess history of drug misuse (Cantrill et al., 2012; Chou, Fanciullo, et al., 2009; Manchikanti et al., 2012a, 2012b; Thorson et al., 2013); however, these guidelines were based mainly on consensus panel recommendations (Cantrill et al., 2012).

Also, we found that the current DoD and VA guidelines regarding substance use discuss general approaches to treatment and are usually not focused on specific management of PDM (Management of

Substance Use Disorders Work Group, 2009). The problem of opioid abuse is particularly challenging, given the need to balance the benefits of pain management and the risk of addiction (Prescription Drug Abuse Subcommittee, 2013).

The five consensus statements all came from the civilian sector: four from the Substance Abuse and Mental Health Services Administration (SAMHSA) (SAMHSA, 2004, 2008, 2009, 2012) and one from the National Institute on Drug Abuse (National Institute on Drug Abuse, 2012). They outlined two main treatment modalities based on expert panel review and synopsis of the literature: pharmacotherapy and behavioral therapy. Evidence-based effective pharmacotherapies include methadone maintenance programs, buprenorphine (with or without naloxone), and naltrexone. Evidence-based behavioral therapies for stimulant and opioid abuse transferable to prescription drug abuse included cognitive behavioral therapy, the Matrix model, and contingency management. The Matrix model is an intensive outpatient treatment approach that incorporates relapse-prevention groups, education groups, social-support groups, individual counseling, and urine and breath testing (Rawson, Shoptaw, et al., 1995; Rawson, Marinelli-Casey, et al., 2004). The intensity of either of these treatments should be based on patient assessment; however, no specific assessment tool was consistently recommended across consensus statements.

We examined seven published systematic reviews referenced in CPGs and consensus statements addressing PDM prevention and treatment (Chapman et al., 2010; Fishbain et al., 2008; Martell et al., 2007; Morasco et al., 2011; Noble et al., 2008; Starrels et al., 2010; Turk, Swanson, and Gatchel, 2008). These reviews were consistent with the recommendations found in the aforementioned guidelines regarding lack of evidence supporting any particular screening instruments or the use of urine drug testing for identifying patients with PDM (SAMHSA, 2009, 2012; Turk, Swanson, and Gatchel, 2008). These reviews generally supported the use of a patient history on illicit-drug use in combination with any single screening instrument (Fishbain et al., 2008; Martell et al., 2007; Morasco et al., 2011; Noble et al., 2008; Turk, Swanson, and Gatchel, 2008).

Systematic Review of Original Studies in the Research Literature

Finally, we conducted a systematic review of original research literature identifying effective prevention and treatment strategies. The main prescription drugs of interest were opioids (morphine, codeine, hydrocodone, oxycodone, methadone, fentanyl, and meperidine), stimulants (methylphenidate, dextroamphetamine with amphetamine), benzodiazepines, and barbiturates. We used Preferred Reporting Items for Systematic Reviews and Meta-Analyses, an international recognized systematic-review method, to guide this process (Moher et al., 2009). To identify articles, we searched for a key words in the following databases: Cochrane Database of Systematic Reviews, Cumulative Index to Nursing and Allied Health Literature, EconLit, Embase, Google Scholar, MEDLINE, PsycINFO, PubMed, Scopus, Sociological Abstracts (ProQuest), and Web of Science. Appendix A provides a comprehensive description of key terms used for this search. We entered a standardized search query into each database. We searched for articles published between 2000 and 2012 in English and involving humans (rather than animal studies).

We reviewed the titles and abstracts of all articles identified through this process for relevance (see Figure 2.1 for a schematic of the article screening and review process). As part of this screening process, we sorted articles as pertaining to either prevention or treatment. We defined *prevention* as efforts helping to identify, educate, or screen those who were not yet experiencing problems related to misuse, while *treatment* refers to services rendered to address and treat those experiencing misuse. The team identified nine articles on PDM prevention and five articles on PDM treatment suitable for data extraction (Baehren et al., 2010; Banta-Green et al., 2009; Blondell et al., 2010; Buelow, Haggard, and Gatchel, 2009; Deitz, Cook, and Hendrickson, 2011; Ilgen et al., 2011; Knisely et al., 2008; Looby and Earleywine, 2010; Potter et al., 2010; Reifler et al., 2012; Sigmon et al., 2009; M. Smith et al., 2008; R. Smith et al., 2010; Weiss et al., 2011).

From this review of the original empirical literature, we discovered few studies addressing the specific problem of PDM, similar to the

Figure 2.1
How We Selected Studies for Systematic Review of Published Research on the Prevention and Treatment of Prescription Drug Misuse

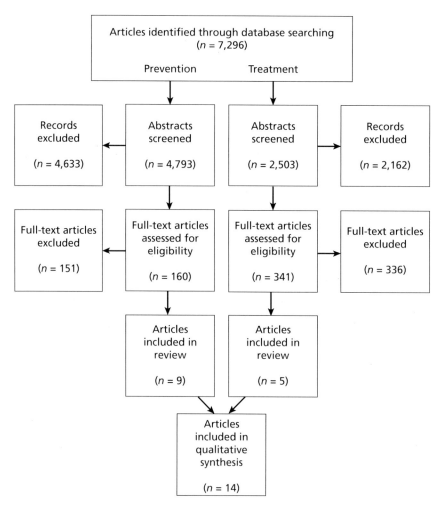

guideline and review literature searches. A few studies have evaluated prevention strategies carefully (Baehren et al., 2010; Buelow, Haggard, and Gatchel, 2009; Deitz, Cook, and Hendrickson, 2011; Ilgen et al., 2011; Knisely et al., 2008; Looby and Earleywine, 2010; Reifler et al.,

2012; M. Smith et al., 2008; R. Smith et al., 2010). However, of the four screening-tool validation studies (Buelow, Haggard, and Gatchel, 2009; Ilgen et al., 2011; Knisely et al., 2008; Looby and Earleywine, 2010; R. Smith et al., 2010), each examined a different instrument to assess opioid misuse. We found only three studies focused on monitoring PDM, and only one of those was quasi-experimental. We identified only one study focused on a behavioral prevention program. A limited number of articles focused specifically on treatment of PDM and prescription drug dependence (Banta-Green et al., 2009; Blondell et al., 2010; Potter et al., 2010; Sigmon et al., 2009; Weiss et al., 2011), all of which focused on short-term treatment. Only some of these studies evaluated practice guidelines for PDM and prescription drug dependence or employed a randomized controlled trial, and none of them used a military population sample.

Conclusions

With the rise in opioid misuse, both the civilian and military medical communities have increased attention to addressing the issue of prescription opioids (Bray, Olmstead, and William, 2012; IOM, 2012; Office of the Army Surgeon General, 2010; SAMHSA, 2002; Prescription Drug Abuse Subcommittee, 2013). The majority of current guidelines, consensus statements, and published literature focus mainly on opioid abuse and note a general lack of evidence of many of the approaches commonly used in practice to predict misuse. Few studies address prevention or treatment approaches. More research is needed to identify and recommend effective mechanisms for addressing the problem of PDM, an issue that is likely to affect both civilian and military populations in decades to come. Given the general lack of evidence base supporting any clear guidelines in the prevention or treatment of PDM, it might be more useful to identify current prevention, identification, and treatment practices in medical treatment facilities than to adhere to specific CPGs. The reviewed DoD policies provided little specific guidance pertaining to PDM and complex language that emphasized zero tolerance approaches to drug abuse over limited-use policies.

CHAPTER THREE

Designing a Tool to Assist in Identifying Prescription Drug Misuse Among Current and Future Active-Duty Service Members

To assist the military in its effort to better understand the extent to which PDM stems from overuse or misuse of medically needed prescriptions versus nonmedical abuse, we developed an analytic tool. Once populated with data available to the military, this tool should be able to assist military commanders in identifying the dynamics of the current PDM problem and develop expectations of how it could change going forward given changes in the demographics of the ADSM population, as well as changes in injury rates associated with military engagements and training. This analytic tool should also provide useful information to military medical personnel about how changes in the identification of PDM and effectiveness of treatment in the military medical sector might influence rates of PDM.

The analytic tool that we developed, described in detail in Appendix B, is commonly referred to as a compartmental model because it breaks up a specific population (in this case, the ADSM population) into different groups (referred to in the model as compartments), which are determined by a common set of conditions that apply to everyone who is placed into the same compartment. The compartmental model is made dynamic by allowing people to transition from compartment to compartment based on a set of rules, typically determined through empirical analysis of available data that form the basis of the rule.

In our analytic tool, the general population of ADSMs is subdivided into 11 groups (or compartments) based on three possible starting points: (1) those who are susceptible to becoming dependent on prescription drugs because of an injury or other medical indication;

(2) those who are susceptible to becoming problem prescription drug users but have no medical need for the drug; and (3) those who are nonsusceptible, meaning those who are not injured and have no risk of becoming nonmedical users. Figure 3.1, which represents a simplified version of the compartmental model that forms the basis of the analytic tool, shows these three starting compartments in green. We use

Figure 3.1
The Compartmental Model as a Basis for the Analytic Tool

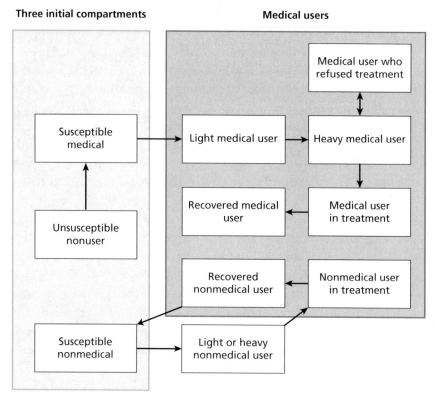

NOTE: The green section indicates how the population of new ADSMs starts in the model, before any military duty takes place. The blue section encompasses users who initiate prescription drug use for medical reasons. Someone is considered to get medical treatment when entering treatment and hence become part of the medical system. Moreover, some people can become addicted to the opioid replacement therapy (e.g., methadone).
RAND RR1345-3.1

the green color is used to indicate how the population of new ADSMs start in the model, before any military duty even takes place. We placed those who are susceptible, either medically or nonmedically, in the user category once prescription drug use is identified. Those who use initially because of a medical indication are easily identifiable within the military TRICARE data (indicated in blue in Figure 3.1). Those who initiate use without a medical need are not identifiable in the health system but should be identified through either self-reports from the Health Related Behaviors Survey (HRBS) or positive drug tests.

In addition to these three compartments, we further categorize the population of medical users in terms of (1) light and heavy use, to capture two different levels of use of prescription drugs; (2) whether those who have access medically refuse treatment or go to treatment; and (3) among those who go to treatment (as a medical or nonmedical user), the stage of treatment they are in—namely, the withdrawal stage (i.e., actually in treatment and going through withdrawals) or a recovered and abstinent stage. Although these categories are obvious oversimplifications, the empirical evidence base on which to more precisely define additional compartments is too limited at this point to support further refinement.

It is possible, through a linked version of the drug testing data and TRICARE medical and pharmacy claim data, to empirically identify the share of the ADSM population that falls into most of the compartments identified in Figure 3.1, particularly those that are part of the MHS. For example, data within TRICARE (including claims submitted from nongovernment personnel) can be used to identify (1) the proportion of people who are receiving a potentially addictive prescription drug, (2) the proportion who are being prescribed relatively high or low doses, and (3) the proportion who are currently in treatment for PDM problems. ADSMs who have successfully completed treatment and are no longer receiving potentially addictive prescriptions for medical indications would represent the recovered population (either medical or nonmedical, depending on whether they were ever provided the prescription that they abused and caused them to need treatment).

Two particular compartments, however, will be difficult to populate (in terms of identifying the share of ADSMs who fall into this category) based on available data: (1) the group of truly unsusceptible users (i.e., people who have no predisposing risk of using a prescription drug nonmedically and have no medical indication for it) and (2) the group who are misusing prescription drugs who have been prescribed them but are currently avoiding treatment, either by hiding their misuse from their medical providers or by not seeking any treatment. In both of these cases, we can construct preliminary estimates. In the case of the first group (i.e., truly unsusceptible users), it might be possible to crosswalk data from HRBS (i.e., those who have never been prescribed a prescription that is commonly abused[1] and never self-report use) with information from drug testing and medical claim data to build a model of the likelihood that someone is not at risk (conditioned on age, for example). Then a prediction model, based on characteristics in these data sets, can be used to generate an estimate of the share of the ADSMs who are truly not susceptible. In the case of the second group (i.e., misusing prescription drugs but avoiding treatment), expert opinion based on interviews with providers who manage patients receiving prescriptions of high abuse potential might be useful. Alternatively, an empirical prediction model using TRICARE pharmacy claim data could be constructed that predicts the likelihood an ADSM (with given characteristics, such as gender, age, or race) is dependent on a drug based on the amount being prescribed to that patient and the duration of the use.

The dynamics of the model, which capture how the share of the population in each of these compartments move from category to category over time, is driven by empirically based transition (change) rules (formally described as differential mathematic equations) based on existing data that represent a modification of the simple mover–stayer drug-use epidemic model presented in Rossi, 2002, and is consistent with other drug using models, as well as models of noninfectious diseases (Everingham and Rydell, 1994; Rydell, Caulkins, and Everingham, 1996; Shallenberger, 1998; Behrens, Caulkins, Tragler, Haunschmied, et al., 1999). These transition rules make use of information available

---

[1]   Some prescription drugs are never abused (e.g., prescription acne cream), while other prescription drugs can be abused if used in excess of recommended doses (e.g., opioids).

through military-specific data sources on average transitions in the current ADSM population. For example, we could model the transition of ADSM from the susceptible-user state to the medical-user state based on rates of injury (caused in combat or in training) requiring prescriptions of abuse.[2] Similarly, we could describe the transition of ADSMs from the heavy-use stage to treatment or withdrawal based on current referral rates to treatment as indicated in the TRICARE data. The dynamics for all of the transitions identified in the model should be feasibly constructed from linked data that military experts have generated in the past (e.g., Jeffery, May, et al., 2014).

Once the dynamics of the compartmental model are determined using information available to the military, the analytic tool will be fully operational and can be used to describe not just the current state of PDM among ADSMs but the dynamics of this misuse. Moreover, it can be used to better understand how current trends in prescription drug availability and prescriptions, the rate of injury, and current demographics of ADSMs translate into future prevalence rates of PDM in the future (i.e., forecasting). We have explicitly designed the analytic tool to forecast how the incidence and prevalence of PDM will change in the future if current practices change or continue with current trends simply by changing the assumed transition rules or rates of identification of specific types of people in a given compartment. For example, the analytic tool can be used to project how PDM might change with a change in initiation rates of light prescription drug use among medical or nonmedical users, changes in escalation rates from light to heavy use, changes in the rate at which people enter treatment, or changes in the relative effectiveness of treatment (i.e., predictive forecasting). Alternatively, the analytic tool could be structured so that all the transition rules and population sizes are specific to a particular class of pre-

---

[2] A susceptible user is someone who might or might not ever be prescribed a prescription opioid. They might just go on to use it without their own prescription (e.g., Ritalin, which those without attention deficit hyperactivity disorder commonly abuse to stay awake for multiple days in a row). We are trying to identify people who are susceptible to misusing a drug (whether it was prescribed to them or not) from those who will never do something that is illegal (too law abiding to do anything wrong—and the military definitely has these types, according to the surveys).

scription drugs (e.g., narcotics, stimulants, or benzodiazepines). A version of the tool that is specific to a particular prescription drug of abuse could enable military health providers to better understand the risks of overprescribing, and hence increasing access to, those particular classes of prescription drugs and generate information that might be useful in educating providers about the risks of overprescribing or not reducing prescribed amounts over time.

The analytic tool that we developed has several limitations, of course. In particular, it relies on simplifying behavioral and biological assumptions about the prescription drug epidemic. Behaviorally, we assume, individuals' transition rates from one PDM state to another can be described by population-level averages, and we assume that people do not influence each other's drug use behavior. Biologically, we assume, everyone in the model has the same escalation risk to PDM once they initiate consumption of a prescription drug, either medically or nonmedically, which is likely to be an oversimplification.[3] Genetic research today clearly shows that people have different genetic dispositions toward alcohol and smoking dependence, and similar genetic differences probably exist with respect to prescription drugs. However, without clearer empirical evidence providing better information on the variability in susceptibility the population, and more critically among the active-duty military population, these sorts of refinements to the model can only add noise and make it harder for the model to reproduce historical data.

A perhaps more significant limitation of the analytic tool is that the compartmental model on which it is based will only reflect information on what is visible or quantifiable in military data sets. Aspects of the PDM problem that are unmeasured, such as the extent to which prescriptions are obtained through outside service providers with no medical claim to TRICARE or drug treatment received outside of the MHS. It might be possible to test assumptions regarding the extent to which these unknowns might be happening, by adjusting the size of

---

[3] This assumption can easily be relaxed, by considering a set of models each with the same structure but with different model parameter values that can represent different population demographics.

the populations in particular compartments or the rates of transition from light medical to heavy medical use. But there will be no way to verify these numbers, and hence no basis on which strong policy recommendations can be made regarding their influence on results obtained from the analytic tool.

Although limited in the ways just mentioned, similar simplified compartmental models have been demonstrated to be highly effective at modeling the population dynamics of other drug use epidemics (Rydell, Caulkins, and Everingham, 1996; Behrens, Caulkins, Tragler, Haunschmied, et al., 1999). Thus, we believe that this strategy could be similarly effective here and adjustments, post–tool development, can be made to capture missing populations, as has been done for heavy drug users in the past. However, like that of all epidemiological models of health behaviors, the value of the analytic tool we propose here will still depend on the reliability of estimates obtained from the data sources available to the military and the quality of the assumptions made regarding information that is missing. Our scan of the data fields contained in the TRICARE, DoD HRBS, and military drug testing data suggest that sufficient information exists to fully describe the model empirically and calculate the transition rules that the tool requires. Standard techniques for checking reliability and validity of the output from the tool using these data would be necessary, but, assuming that the tool is shown to be both externally valid and reliable, the tool proposed here could provide military leadership with guidance on how to target limited prevention and treatment dollars toward the key factors that appear to drive higher rates of misuse in the overall ADSM population.

CHAPTER FOUR

Our Qualitative Assessment of Military Health Providers' Views on Prescription Drug Misuse

Introduction

The final task we conducted was the implementation of qualitative interviews with medical health providers, including emergency room (ER) doctors, physicians, nurses, physician assistants (PAs), case managers, social workers, mental health therapists, pain medicine specialists, substance abuse treatment providers, and pharmacists, across nine medical treatment facility (MTFs). Our goals of these interviews were threefold: (1) to assess the extent to which providers perceive PDM as a problem among ADSMs; (2) to better understand provider awareness and implementation of CPGs and DoD policies pertaining to PDM; and (3) to hear what providers view as challenges in the identification, management, and treatment of PDM among ADSMs and what sort of recommendations they had for overcoming these challenges.

Although a recent IOM report on substance use disorders (SUDs) in the military (IOM, 2012) provided a comprehensive assessment of current DoD policies for identifying and treating substance abuse among ADSMs and offered several useful recommendations for improvement, the report does not examine policies and practices for addressing PDM specifically. Evidence-based interventions and treatments for preventing and treating PDM are few (Blanchard et al., 2016), but there is some evidence supporting the use of screening tools to assess the potential for misuse, as well as behavioral and pharmacological treatments for opioid dependence. There are also DoD policies and instructions (DoDD 1010.1 [Assistant Secretary of Defense for Special Operations and Low-Intensity Conflict, 1999a], DoDD 1010.4

[Assistant Secretary of Defense for Special Operations and Low-Intensity Conflict, 1999b], DoDI 1010.6 [Assistant Secretary of Defense for Health Affairs, 1985]) for managing SUDs, VA/DoD CPGs for addressing SUDs and pain (Management of Substance Use Disorders Work Group, 2009; Management of Opioid Therapy for Chronic Pain Working Group, 2010; Chou, Qaseem, et al., 2007), and service-specific programs and policies related to treatment (AFI 44-121 [Deputy Surgeon General of the Air Force, 2011], AR 600-85 [Headquarters, Department of the Army, 2012b], BUMEDINST 5350.4D [Director, Personal Readiness and Community Support Branch, 2009], Marine Corps Order 5300.17 [Deputy Commandant for Manpower and Reserve Affairs, 2011]). To assess the implementation of DoD policies and CPGs specific to PDM and to learn about innovative practices, as well as implementation barriers across the service branches, we conducted individual face-to-face interviews with 66 health and behavioral health providers at nine MTFs across three regions between July and November 2014. The regions were those identified through TRICARE pharmacy data as high or average prescribing areas for opioids and benzodiazepines, two drugs of high abuse in the military. We interviewed physicians from primary care and family medicine practices, as well as ER physicians, nurses and PAs, pain specialists, mental and behavioral health providers, pharmacists, case managers, and SUD treatment providers.

In this chapter, we describe our methods for identifying MTFs and health providers, as well as the interview protocol used in the conduct of the interviews. We also discuss the limitations of the methods we used in terms of our ability to draw broad policy recommendations from this, which is important when considering the recommendations that providers made later in the chapter.

All data-collection procedures were submitted to and approved by the RAND Human Subjects Protection Committee, the Office of the Assistant Secretary of Defense for Health Affairs, and the Department of the Navy Human Research Protection Program; all deemed the procedures exempt from committee review. Washington Headquarters Service also approved procedures. The interview guide was approved by Defense Manpower Data Center and given a report control symbol: DDHA(A)2553.

Methods

Recruitment and Participants

We began by identifying regions of the country in which high levels of opioid and benzodiazepine prescription drugs are being prescribed to ADSMs and their family members, as indicated by TRICARE outpatient pharmacy data from 2010 (see Table 4.1). We identified opi-

Table 4.1
Opioid and Benzodiazepine Prescriptions in TRICARE Pharmacy Data in the Contiguous United States, 2010, as Percentages

Region	Opioid Prescriptions	Benzodiazepine Prescriptions	Total Prescriptions
Northeast	2.21	0.79	11.24
Mid-Atlantic	2.32	1.06	12.65
Southeast	2.53	1.02	11.13
Gulf Coast	2.61	1.22	5.90
Heartland	2.37	1.21	8.56
Southwest	2.56	0.91	12.56
Central	2.58	1.01	14.00
West, Southern California	2.21	0.87	6.28
West, Golden Gate	2.54	1.17	1.85[a]
Northwest	2.88	0.91	4.07

SOURCE: Our analysis of 2010 TRICARE pharmacy data.

[a] Frequently, opioids are prescribed *with* benzodiazepines (in combination), so they are often *not* the sum of the two. Moreover, the total number of prescriptions is the summary of the number of per capita prescriptions of any prescription drug—not just these two—and it turns out that the West, Golden Gate, region is very low in prescribing.

ates and benzodiazepines in the pharmacy data using both the therapeutic class names (280,808 for opiates and 282,408 for diazepines) and product names. The specific opiates of interest were hydrocodone, oxycodone, codeine, propoxyphene, morphine, hydromorphone, fentanyl, oxymorphone, meperidine, levorphanol, and dihydrocodeine. The specific benzodiazepines of interest included diazepam (Valium or Diastat), alprazolam (Xanax or Niravam), lorazepam (Ativan), and chlordiazepoxide (Librium).

Table 4.1 shows the prevalence of prescriptions for opioids, benzodiazepines, and any prescription drug by region where beneficiaries live for those ADSMs living within the contiguous United States. The regions are the standard regions specified in military data. The table shows that, although only 4 percent of all prescriptions were written in the Northwest region, the rate of prescribing a prescription opiate there was the highest for all U.S. regions. The rate for prescribing benzodiazepines was on the lower side, however. The Gulf Coast region had a fairly low percentage of total prescriptions but had the highest rate of benzodiazepine prescribing and relatively high rate of opioid prescribing. Thus, we automatically considered installations within these two regions for inclusion in the sampling frame because they anchored the maximum rate of prescriptions across all regions.

Southern California had a relatively low rate of both opioid and benzodiazepine prescribing but also a relatively low total prescription rate overall. We included it in the sample because it suggested to us that military providers in this region might be more cautious than average at prescribing anything. Finally, we sought to include a region that had generally higher rates of prescribing any prescription overall. We selected the mid-Atlantic region because we knew that (1) it had several treatment facilities that focused on substance abuse and (2) it showed good diversity in terms of military branches represented in the region.

After picking broad regions based on basic prescribing patterns observed in the TRICARE pharmacy data, we selected a purposive convenience sample of MTFs within each region that represented different types of MTFs, different sizes of facilities, and different service branches (see Table 4.2). We originally contacted 12 MTFs; 11 responded, and we were able to schedule interviews at nine. We then

Table 4.2
Descriptive Information on the Facilities Selected to Participate in Our Study

Facility	Region	State	Facility Type	Facility Size	Service Branch
1	Mid-Atlantic	Virginia	Health clinic	Small	Army
2			Hospital or outpatient clinic	Small	Air Force
3	Gulf Coast	Florida	Hospital or outpatient clinic	Medium	Navy and Marine Corps
4			Health clinic	Small	Air Force
5			Hospital or outpatient clinic	Medium	Air Force
6		Texas	Medical center	Small	Army
7		Texas	Medical center	Large	Army
8	Southern California	California	Medical center	Large	Navy and Marine Corps
9	Northwest	Washington	Medical center satellite health clinic	Small	Air Force

NOTE: Small < 50,000 patients served. Medium = 50,000–99,999. Large ≥ 100,000.

emailed the commander of each MTF and requested a point of contact (POC). Appendix C provides a sample email. The commanders forwarded our email requests to the POCs, and we followed up by email and then, in most cases, by telephone.

We identified providers through a self-selection process. We asked each POC to announce the study to a variety of provider types (e.g., ER, primary care and family physicians, pain specialists, nurses and PAs, case managers, pharmacists, mental health therapists, and SUD treatment specialists) and to request volunteers to sign up for 45-minute to one-hour face-to-face interviews. We provided language for the POCs to use in their emails to providers and emphasized that the participation was voluntary. We confirmed the voluntary nature of the study in person immediately prior to conducting interviews and offered volunteers the opportunity to decline participation. Every volunteer who came for an interview appointment elected to participate.

Sixty-six volunteers across nine MTFs participated in the study. Unfortunately, we could not obtain information on the number of actual practitioners, overall or by type, who worked in any of our nine MTFs. Thus, we do not know the extent to which the sample we obtained is representative of either all treatment providers or those engaged in delivering substance abuse treatment. However, we can say that many providers who self-selected to participate were relatively knowledgeable about the treatment of ADSMs believed to be suffering with PDM. Prior to the interviews, we described the study in detail and obtained spoken consent of each medical provider to participate in the research. Participants represented 13 professions and specialties (see Table 4.3). We cannot provide details of participating providers by MTF because doing so might risk identification of a participant or specific MTF in the study.

Interview Protocol and Data-Collection Procedures

We created a discussion guide that addressed general impressions of PDM among ADSMs; policies, practices, and training; experiences, challenges, and barriers; and recommendations (see Appendix C). Interviews were semistructured, individual, and face to face and were conducted at each installation MTF. Two RAND researchers conducted each interview; one was the primary interviewer, and the other researcher took notes. The interviewing researcher used the guide to steer the conversation, probe for additional information, and ensure that all domains were covered; the interview was not administered as a structured, question-by-question interview.

Upon completion of the interviews, the two researchers independently categorized all provider comments from each interview into the primary domains in the discussion guide: provider perspectives; policies and practices for preventing, identifying, and treating PDM; training availability, participation, and needs; and challenges and recommendations. Following initial, independent categorization, the researchers reconciled their coding discrepancies and formed a consensus regarding the categorization of themes. The researchers then

Table 4.3
Types of Military Health Providers Who Agreed to Participate in Our Study

Profession	Specialization	N
Case manager		8
Mental health	Psychology or psychiatry	3
Registered nurse, NP, or PA		13
Physician	ER	7
	Family medicine	6
	Other (medical director, chief medical officer, or internal medicine)	3
	Primary care	3
	Pain specialist	6
Pharmacist	General	6
	Clinical	4
Substance abuse treatment specialist (counselor, psychologist, or psychiatrist)		7
Total		66

NOTE: NP = nurse practitioner.

reviewed all comments and placed them into subcategories. For example, within the domain of policies and practices for preventing PDM, subcategories included sole-provider (SP) and other medication-related agreements, assessments and screening tools, refill policies and practices, medication reconciliation and monitoring, and interdisciplinary coordination.[1] We reviewed each domain and subcategory for common elements and themes. In this report, we present modal themes, as well as key points and the diverse array of perspectives and practices that emerged from the analysis. Because this study did not involve a random sample of sites within regions and branches, a nonrandom sample of

---

[1] Medication reconciliation is a process in which a provider and patient review a comprehensive list of all active and former medications the patient has been prescribed.

providers within sites (because providers volunteered), and a nonrandom sample of regions, we do not systematically report on differences by region, service branch, MTF or provider type, except where salient differences emerged and MTFs and providers would not be identified.

Findings fall into the following categories:

- provider perspectives on the nature and extent of PDM among ADSMs
- DoD, MTF, and clinic-level policies and practices for preventing, identifying, managing, and treating PDM
- training availability, participation, and needs
- provider perspectives on challenges to effectively managing PDM and recommendations for improving prevention, identification, and treatment of PDM.

Limitations of Our Approach

Although we obtained rich and detailed data from selected providers of different types within these nine MTFs, we note several limitations of the study. First, we base the insights and recommendations on a nonrandom sample of providers within a nonrandom sample of MTFs. Because of our limited budget, we selected MTFs so as to maximize the likelihood that providers would encounter PDM users, based on the number of prescriptions written in that general region in a previous year. Moreover, not all MTFs selected based on region and prescribing patterns responded to our request to interview providers. Thus, we did not randomly or even probabilistically select the MTFs.

Similarly, providers within MTFs were not a random sample but rather reflected a convenience sample of those providers who volunteered to participate in the study once either the MTF commander or our interview team made them aware of it. Between six and eight providers at each site self-selected to participate in an interview; at some sites, not all provider types were represented. More importantly, because we do not know the exact number of providers of each type working at each MTF, we do not know the extent to which those who participated represent a small or large proportion of providers of a given type.

Third, the interviews were semistructured, meaning that some providers chose to focus more on some topics than others. As such, findings from these interviews, although valuable, should be interpreted with caution. Practices within MTFs might extend beyond what providers in this study reported, and practices and perspectives might be different among providers with whom we did not speak and in regions we did not visit.

These limitations notwithstanding, the voices and opinions heard during the course of this study are not inconsistent or significantly different from those raised in nonmilitary samples, according to our literature review, which were similarly focused on issues related to resources, electronic medical records (EMRs), and access to state PDMPs.

Findings

Provider's Perceptions of Prescription Drug Misuse Among Active-Duty Service Members

Participating providers across the nine MTFs shared their perspectives on the nature and extent of PDM among ADSMs. Despite differences in the types of military health providers interviewed, the service branches that the MTFs represented, and the types of medical facilities in which we conducted our interviews, key themes emerged in terms of the participating providers' perceptions of the PDM problem. Table 4.4 provides an overview of the key themes among participating providers, and the rest of this chapter provides more-detailed discussion of these themes.

Providers Agreed That Prescription Drug Misuse Is a Problem

Although many military health providers across MTFs and provider types noted that ADSMs are held to a higher standard than civilians and that the military has more protocols in place for preventing PDM, including substantially greater consequences, most providers interviewed generally agreed that there is indeed a PDM problem that must

Table 4.4
Overview of Participating Providers' Perspectives on the Nature and Extent of Prescription Drug Misuse

Category	Perspective
Participating providers across military treatment facilities believe that PDM is a problem.	PDM is present in all service branches, but airmen (Air Force service members) might experience slightly less PDM because of stringent flight regulations.
	Interviewees reported on three types of misuse—misuse due to medically indicated pain; misuse due to medically indicated pain that turns into misuse that continues after pain has subsided; and misuse with no medically indicated origin. Most PDM among ADSMs originates from some form of medically indicated use.
	Purchasing medication outside of the MHS is believed to be difficult to track and presents a serious problem to military health providers.
	Purely nonmedical use of prescription medications occurs but is not thought to be common practice among ADSMs.
Providers perceive opioids to be the most commonly misused prescription drug.	A variety of opioids (e.g., Percocet [oxycodone with acetaminophen], Vicodin [hydrocodone with acetaminophen], Lortab [hydrocodone], Dilaudid [hydromorphone]) were reported as the most commonly misused prescription drugs.
	Stimulants, such as Adderall, also might be misused among airmen (more than other ADSMs) because of requirements to maintain concentration for long periods of time.
	Sleep medications are also misused but perceived as less frequently a problem.
PDM is perceived to be due to a variety of provider, patient, and cultural factors.	Perceived provider factors include provider prescribing practices; lack of training or expertise, time, and resources; and inconsistencies in the implementation of policies and procedures.
	Perceived patient factors include lack of patients' education about their prescription medications and psychological vulnerability of personnel who have been in combat or injured in training.
	Perceived cultural factors include pain treatment that is currently thought of as clinically appropriate in the medical community but might not be optimal or sustainable for patients, as well as the definition of *misuse* and the consequences and stigma related to it, which might affect treatment for and recovery from PDM.

Table 4.4—Continued

Category	Perspective
PDM is perceived to be more common among family members of ADSMs than among ADSMs themselves.	Interviewees reported that dependents who present in MTFs have been to multiple doctors over many years, some of them from locations across the country and overseas.
	Some dependents might actively seek medications and doctor-shop and receive medications that get diverted to them from ADSMs.

be addressed and that PDM among ADSMs mirrors PDM in the civilian population. According to providers, reasons that ADSMs might misuse prescription drugs despite potentially severe consequences (i.e., administrative separation from the military) include their high susceptibility to injury, the medically indicated need for prescription pain medication, and the iatrogenic dependence that can result from the use of opioid pain medications. As one NP noted, "One can become legitimately dependent on opioids, but it's when it gets to the doctor-shopping or harm that it becomes a problem."

Perceptions of the extent of misuse varied slightly across service branches, with providers who treat active-duty Air Force personnel noting that airmen might misuse less because of more-stringent regulations for flying than for engaging in other military activities and perceptions of a stricter zero tolerance policy.

Providers perceived several different types of misuse among ADSMs. An ADAPT counselor summarized three types of PDM this way:

> I think [that PDM] is a pretty significant issue. I do separate the three types [of misuse] out in my mind. One is that you're in legitimate pain and have been prescribed a medication and, as time rolls on, there are pain management interventions being provided but ultimately leading to greater pain medication use. I've had some people who have recognized their own burgeoning dependence. There are others with legitimate pain issues [who] are abusing and becoming dependent and eventually reaching out and seeking more—your doctor-shoppers, those who use their wife's prescriptions, those who substitute with more illicit drugs.

Then there are those [who] have no legitimate use or prescriptions for these medications who are accessing [them] along with other drugs.

Providers generally agreed that the most common type of misuse occurs among ADSMs who initially receive a medically indicated prescription for acute or chronic pain and then develop a dependence on the medication because of the same, possibly worsening, medical issue or they continue taking it for other reasons, such as self-medicating to deal with emotional issues or other types of physical pain. This might lead to drug-seeking behaviors and doctor-shopping. Most providers are well aware of drug-seeking behaviors, which include ADSMs coming in for their refills too soon, claiming they lost their prescriptions, or asking for a specific medication and sometimes claiming they are allergic to all others. Doctor-shopping also occurs, with ADSMs going to the ER for extra medication or seeking additional prescriptions from a variety of doctors within the MTF or from civilian physicians outside of the MTF.

Providers across all MTFs stated that purchasing medication outside of the MHS presents a serious problem because medications purchased with cash, instead of through TRICARE health insurance, cannot be tracked in the Armed Forces Health Longitudinal Technology Application (AHLTA) Composite Health Care System (CHCS), the primary military EMR system. Some providers noted that EMRs within and across installations do not typically share information, which increases the opportunity for drug-seeking ADSMs to "game" the system. A registered nurse made the following observation: "I'm sure there are active-duty personnel [who] can get the pain medication they want through various means, whether it is a dentist, an [ear, nose, and throat doctor] or a PCP [primary care physician]."

Most providers do not think that overtly nonmedical use of prescription medication (i.e., taking pills just to get high) is common among ADSMs, although providers admitted that they might not be privy to information about such practices. One pharmacist noted once hearing about "trail mix," a practice in which ADSMs pool their prescription pills in a bag and then share the pills with other ADSMs to get high, but did not think that this was currently a common practice. A nurse provided this anecdote: "At my last base, everyone had to be drug screened because someone with a legitimate Percocet prescription was just handing it out to people." Another nurse noted that this type of behavior was more of a problem in the past than it is now:

> In the barracks, at one time, there was tons of "Percocet poker" and trading and sharing . . . but now, in the barracks, there are military wellness and health inspections and monitoring posts that have largely made it more difficult to be trading and sharing medications in the barracks.

Although providers do not perceive nonmedical use as common, a few providers expressed concerns about diversion. Some mentioned possible diversion to family members, while others mentioned diversion in the form of selling or bartering. A physician provided this anecdote:

> I'm seeing a lot of diversion in the military; there's street value in [the medications]. This is why it's so important to drug screen the soldiers, which I do routinely. I will have patients on opiates, and they will fool me, primarily for diversion. And they may not be selling the drugs; they may be giving it to the wife or family member with a pain problem. This guy was on Percocet for a herniated disk and screened negative twice on the urinary drug screen. I was shocked.

Opioids Are the Most Commonly Misused Prescription Drugs

Almost all providers said that opioid pain medications are the most misused prescription medications, though misused brands vary slightly across regions and facilities. Most providers reported that oxycodone (e.g., Oxycontin) or hydrocodone (e.g., Zohydro ER) alone or in combination, such as Percocet (e.g., oxycodone with acetaminophen) or Vicodin, Norco, and Lortab (e.g., hydrocodone with acetaminophen, in varied proportions), were the most frequently misused prescription drugs. Some providers noted that Ultram (brand name of tramadol) was commonly misused because it was not listed or treated as a controlled substance until August 2014. As such, it was frequently prescribed as an alternative to pain medications believed to be addictive and, in turn, it was more commonly misused by ADSMs. Some providers noted that certain service members in specific branches seek stimulants, such as Adderall (in addition to opioids), noting one possible reason as their need to stay alert with heightened reflexes for long periods of time (e.g., pilots). Service providers also noted that sleep medications, such as Ambien, are overprescribed and often misused.

Prescription Drug Misuse Is Due to a Combination of Provider, Patient, and Cultural Factors

Providers across all MTFs believe that a variety of factors contribute to PDM among ADSMs. The most commonly mentioned factors included lack of provider training and expertise in pain management and long-term opioid therapy, overprescribing, lack of provider continuity and consistency in prescribing practices, and lack of time for primary care providers and resources within MTFs to properly manage patients with chronic pain. The patient factors mentioned included ADSMs' lack of understanding of the nature of the medications and how to take them, psychological vulnerability due to trauma, and predisposition to addiction. Cultural factors that some providers mentioned included the "pill culture" that predominates in both military and civilian medical practices and varied philosophies about how to approach pain and pain management.

Provider Factors: Training and Expertise, Time and Resources, and Inconsistency

About 30 percent of the providers in each region mentioned that provider prescribing practices contribute to misuse. Nurses, social workers, and pain specialists whom we interviewed observed that the lack of resources, including lack of referral options for chronic pain patients; the lack of continuity between providers; time and training among primary care managers (PCMs) contributing to their overprescribing pain medications; failing to provide adequate patient education; lack of monitoring and follow-up; and not following CPGs for patients on long-term opioid therapy. Some of these providers also believe that, in some cases, PCMs continue prescribing medication long after patients need it. PCMs (and other physicians), on the other hand, observed that midlevel prescribers, NPs, and PAs are not well trained in managing patients on pain medications but are typically assigned to chronic pain patients when they are referred back to primary care after seeing pain specialists. As one physician noted, "Some midlevel providers have specialty training, but many have not and are not comfortable prescribing large doses of serious narcotics." Many providers—physicians and others—agreed that pain specialists are the best equipped to handle patients with chronic pain because they are well educated in pharmacotherapy and in alternative treatments, but they also noted that there are only enough resources for patients to be seen by specialists for a short period of time, that there is a dearth of these specialists and specialty clinics at MTFs, and that resources for complementary and alternative practices across the military are inadequate to meet the demand. A registered nurse observed inconsistencies in how providers handle chronic pain patients and prescribing pain medications:

> The procedure varies on a case-by-case basis. My providers work a little differently. One of them won't prescribe narcotics over the phone and will refer anyone requiring chronic pain meds to pain management. The other provider will prescribe over the phone and fill prescriptions for one month at a time. She'll see them periodically and do it over the phone.

Patient Factors: Education and Psychological Vulnerability

Some providers whom we interviewed observed that the lack of patient education about the risks of their prescription medications, how to take them, and the consequences of taking them other than prescribed is contributing to PDM. Others noted the psychological vulnerability and thus greater susceptibility to dependence on medication of personnel who have been in combat or injured in training. A nurse said this about patient education:

> I don't think [that] our active-duty population is educated on narcotic use and on the consequences of narcotic use . . . They don't realize that it's not okay to take narcotics six months down the

line after a sprained ankle, as opposed to the pharmacy educating them on the way to use the medication.

A physician put it this way: "A lot of soldiers have not been told that the expectation of their treatment is to minimize pain while making them as functional as possible, not eliminating all pain." A psychologist who works in a pain clinic commented on service member vulnerability:

> The population is comprised of ADSMs who have been injured and have chronic pain problems; in this subpopulation, the incidence of opioid prescribing is higher, as well as the incidence of comorbidities (e.g., traumatic brain injury and posttraumatic stress disorder). These people may also have less robust coping capabilities.

Cultural Factors: Approaches to Pain Management, Definition of *Misuse*, and Stigma

A handful of providers across provider types, including case managers, pain specialists, nurses, and physicians, suggested that the way people think about and treat pain in American culture—in both military and civilian populations—is a factor contributing to PDM among ADSMs. Although providers might be treating patients in a clinically appropriate manner, some noted that treatment currently thought of as clinically appropriate might not be optimal or sustainable for patients. One provider explained his perspective:

> It's great to treat pain, but, even as a military [system], we're not treating it in a wise manner. People are being set up for failure. Giving someone six Percocet and shooing them out of the office isn't the solution. We have all these alternative modalities that no one seems to want; they just want their pills. People have an expectation that pain will be completely removed. There needs to be a change in the way the military deals with opioids. . . . There's still a perception that, if someone has pain, the docs need to treat it and that you'll get in trouble if you don't treat them. We all know that's not the right thing; it'll get them out of your office, but it won't help in the long term if your problem escalates.

Also at issue among some providers is the definition of *misuse* and the consequences and stigma related to it. Patients who currently or who once had chronic pain and become dependent on their medications are quickly stigmatized and thought of as drug users and are treated in a manner similar to ADSMs who use illicit drugs, which could result in administrative separation from the military. Although this might not contribute to misuse per se, providers think that it might affect the treatment patients receive and their recovery from PDM because fear of disciplinary action might prevent ADSMs from seeking access to treatment. In the view of some providers, taking a previously prescribed opioid for a new nonsevere acute injury,[2] even if the medication is past its expiration date, does not warrant the label "PDM" or potential administrative consequences.

Providers Perceive That Prescription Drug Misuse Is Less Common Among Active-Duty Service Members Than Among Those Service Members' Family Members and Spouses

Although the focus of this inquiry was on use among ADSMs, providers at every MTF that we visited commented that, although misuse is a noteworthy problem among ADSMs, they believe that the larger problem is with family members—wives in particular. Very often, multiple doctors have treated a service member's family member who presents in an MTF, some of them from locations across the country and overseas. A physician commented, "The most typical patient I receive is going to be a dependent who has been off the radar, off site, who has seen a candy doctor who has just given them meds after meds after meds." An ER nurse offered his perspective this way:

> The problem is more prevalent amongst dependents . . . seven to eight out of ten patients with these issues are dependents—wives. The most commonly sought-out drugs are morphine and Dilaudid. They want the strongest thing possible. They will tell you that they're allergic to morphine in order to get the stronger stuff. That in and of itself is a red flag.

---

[2] Someone could strain their back and take a medication already in their medicine cabinet, even if their back isn't severe enough to warrant that kind of pain medication.

Some providers discussed family members who were actively seeking medications and doctor-shopping, while others noted that ADSMs sometimes divert the medications to their family members. Of note, research on SUD among dependents of ADSMs is very limited (IOM, 2012).

Awareness of Policies, Clinical Practice Guidelines, and Directives Aimed at Preventing Prescription Drug Misuse

In this section, we present themes that arose when we asked providers about MTF- and clinic-level policies and procedures in place for preventing PDM. Again, despite this being a very limited sample of providers across a small number of MTFs, several interesting and important main themes arose from our interviews about how they perceived the implementation of policies and CPGs that were in place pertaining to substance abuse most generally, but PDM in particular. Here we outline an overview of these key themes related to the *prevention* of PDM, and a detailed discussion of each theme follows:

- Providers perceive SP and high-risk medication agreements as common but inconsistently defined, implemented, documented, and accessed within and across service branches. They also perceive multiple barriers to implementation.
  - Some facilities use agreements for all patients who receive any controlled substances, while others use them for patients perceived as high risk.
  - Agreements are implemented inconsistently within and across MTFs and service branches.
  - Perceived barriers to implementation include the inability to track patients on SP agreements, visits to doctors outside of the MHS, and medications purchased outside the MHS.
- Specialty providers sometimes use standardized assessments to determine potential for PDM, but providers did not report these assessments as regularly administered in general or emergency medicine.
  - The Opioid Risk Tool (Webster and Webster, 2005) and the diagnosis, intractability, risk, and efficacy score (Belgrade,

Schamber, and Lindgren, 2006) are sometimes used to assess patients' risk for opioid abuse.

- The Screener and Opioid Assessment for Patients with Pain— Revised (SOAPP-R) (Butler, Budman, Fernandez, Fanciullo, et al., 2009) is sometimes used to assess how much monitoring a patient will require if the patient is put on opioids.
- The Current Opioid Misuse Measure (COMM) (Butler, Budman, Fernandez, Houle, et al., 2009) is sometimes used to assess whether a patient on opioid therapy is misusing medication.

• Providers use a variety of guidelines and tools for preventing PDM, but the guidelines and tools appear to be inconsistently implemented across MTFs and providers.
- Interviewees noted that some providers use CPGs, but interview data showed that they are used inconsistently and use is not monitored.
- Prescription end dates are thought of as a potential way to deter misuse, but few providers seem to be aware that these are in already use through the MHS.
- Interviewees reported that limitations are placed on dosages, pills, and refills, but implementation is inconsistent, potentially making misuse easier.
- Planned titration frequency was reported as occasional and seldom planned at the outset of chronic opioid therapy.
- Chronic pain, high utilizer, polypharmacy (CHUP) data and risk stratification are used at some Army MTFs but were not reported elsewhere within our sample.
- Clinical pharmacy, case management, and interdisciplinary coordination, when available, appear to greatly facilitate prevention and management of PDM.
- With few exceptions, interviewees did not report medication reconciliation as part of standard clinical care.
- Providers reported referral for complementary and alternative pain management as important parts of treating chronic pain, but resources are few at smaller bases.

- Pill disposal and take-back can occur only through planned take-back events (due to U.S. Drug Enforcement Administration [DEA] regulations); these are generally viewed as very successful.

Agreements Appear Common but Inconsistently Defined and Implemented

Providers across MTFs reported the use of SP or high-risk medication agreements or contracts for preventing PDM among ADSMs. It is important to note that many of the providers with whom we spoke told us that their bases are phasing out the word *contract* in favor of *agreement*; henceforth, in this report, we use the term *agreement*. In general, these agreements limit patients to a single prescribing physician for all medications (i.e., an SP) and might have other requirements regarding refills, frequency of medical appointments, and consequences of misuse (i.e., high-risk medication agreement). Providers also reported that these agreements are inconsistently defined and implemented within and across installations and services and that there are barriers to effectively implementing them (see Table 4.5).

Table 4.5
Examples of Variations in Features, Implementation, and Barriers Reported in Our Qualitative Interviews with Military Providers

Facility	Type of Agreement Cited	Key Features (As Described by Providers)	Implementation	Barrier
1	SP	Single prescriber	Used for people prescribed opioid medications with abuse potential	Referrals to SP are slow and are usually after the PCP determines that the PCP cannot handle the patient any more.
2	SP	Single provider; no early refills; no sharing, selling, or trading	Used for any WTU service member prescribed any controlled substance for >1 month	Not flagged in AHLTA; not routinely implemented

Table 4.5—Continued

Facility	Type of Agreement Cited	Key Features (As Described by Providers)	Implementation	Barrier
3	SP	Single prescriber; single pharmacist	Used for people with "regular periods of medication use"	None reported
4	Pain contract	Single prescriber	Used for potential misusers; used at provider discretion	Inconsistently used by providers
5	Medication and single-prescriber agreement	Single prescriber; no early refills	Used for all patients on any controlled medication beyond one prescription	Single provider is not always available; inconsistent implementation across bases
6	High-risk medication agreement [New]	Option for single provider; random UA; single pharmacy	All providers will use for any patient on pain medication for >2 months; scanned into AHLTA	None
7	Pain contract and medication agreement	Single provider	Used at provider discretion for patients who might benefit	Used inconsistently
8	Pain contract	Single prescriber; UAs at provider discretion	Used for all patients with chronic pain	Inconsistent implementation; provider is not always available; not flagged in AHLTA
9	Opioid agreement	Required UA; multiple patient instructions	Used for all patients on opioids >90 days	Moved away from SP requirement because of team-based practice; not flagged in AHLTA

NOTE: WTU = Warrior Transition Unit. UA = urinalysis.

Agreements typically incorporate assigning patients to a single provider for all of their prescriptions, conducting random urine drug tests ordered at the provider's discretion, educating the patient about the proper use of the medication and the terms of the agreement, and sometimes conducting medication reconciliation, during which a provider and patient review a comprehensive list of all active and former medications a patient has been prescribed. In the context of *preventing* PDM, some facilities use an agreement for every patient who receives any controlled substance, while others use an agreement for any patient perceived as high risk (i.e., taking narcotics for chronic pain, on opioids for more than 60 days, or high service utilizers).

Providers generally agree that the use of agreements is essential to managing medication and preventing misuse, but they also report several barriers to their implementation. Barriers include inconsistent implementation by providers within the same facility and across facilities and bases; difficulty identifying patients on an agreement because of inconsistent documentation and the lack of flags or alerts in AHLTA that are supposed to specifically identify patients on an agreement; inability of some types of providers (e.g., dentists) to identify patients on an agreement or to enter information about them in the EMR because they lack access to AHLTA; inability to efficiently track patients' visits to civilian physicians; and inability to track medications that patients purchase outside of their TRICARE insurance from civilian pharmacies. Patient adherence to agreements also can be an issue. One pharmacist noted,

> [Adherence is] about 50/50. In some cases, [the agreement] opens [the patient's] eyes to the situation; for the other half, it seems like just another formality, and it becomes more for the provider's sake in terms of liability. These also tend to be the [patients who] have been removed from multiple pain clinics. So you're starting off on rough terrain.

Standardized Assessments Are Sometimes Used but Are Not Regularly Administered

According to the providers we interviewed, pain specialists, military SUD treatment providers (ADAPT, the Navy Substance Abuse Rehabilitation Program [SARP], and the Army Substance Abuse Program [ASAP]), and providers serving patients in the WTU sometimes use standardized assessments for potential PDM. However, the providers with whom we spoke said that the assessments are not typically used in general-medicine clinics or in hospitals. If assessments are used at all, they might be used to determine (1) patients' risk for opioid abuse (using such tools as the Opioid Risk Tool [Webster and Webster, 2005] or the diagnosis, intractability, risk, and efficacy score [Belgrade, Schamber, and Lindgren, 2006]); (2) the amount of monitoring a patient will require if put on opioids (using the SOAPP-R [Butler, Budman, Fernandez, Fanciullo, et al., 2009]); and (3) whether patients on opioid therapy are misusing their medication (using the COMM [Butler, Budman, Fernandez, Houle, et al., 2009]).

Although PCMs and other providers working in primary care, family medicine, and ERs do not typically use these standardized risk assessments, they do administer standard tobacco, alcohol, and suicide screeners, as well as subjective pain scale measures. A nurse (among others) expressed the need for better assessments:

> I screen [the patients]. I take their vital signs and document what they tell me. I always ask them if their pain is better, worse, or no change. If worse, I ask them how it's gotten worse, so I can always describe what is going on. We don't always know their history. We do alcohol and tobacco screens but aren't relying on them to be honest. We need more in-depth questions.

A physician also noted that the use of a standardized tool for assessment of misuse among those on opioid therapy would be helpful: "When patients make you uneasy with their general presentation— e.g., [they tell you] 'only Percocet works for me'—it would be better to have a screening tool that doesn't make me rely singularly on intuition." The same physician said that the pain clinic at his MTF introduced the SOAPP-R and the COMM into the family medicine clinic but that the tools were never incorporated into the schedule of regular screenings.

Providers Reported a Variety of Guidelines and Tools

Although providers did not report standardized screeners as administered regularly outside of specialty settings (i.e., pain clinics; drug treatment programs; or specialized programs, such as the WTU), providers reported using CPGs and other tools to prevent misuse. Although these are not consistently used across MTFs and often were reported with disclaimers, most providers are attempting to prevent PDM. In the rest of this section, we describe guidelines and tools that providers reported, as well as provider comments about their implementation.

Clinical Practice Guidelines

Although not all providers reported use of specific CPGs, those specifically mentioned were

- *VA/DoD Clinical Practice Guideline for the Management of Opioid Therapy for Chronic Pain* (Management of Opioid Therapy for Chronic Pain Working Group, 2010)
- "Diagnosis and Treatment of Low Back Pain: A Joint Clinical Practice Guideline from the American College of Physicians and the American Pain Society" (Chou, Qaseem, et al., 2007)
- *VA/DoD Clinical Practice Guideline for Management of Substance Use Disorders* (Management of Substance Use Disorders Work Group, 2009).

Some providers noted that there is poor adherence to CPGs. One pain specialist is helping develop a systemwide (including VA) CPG-adherence program, as well as metrics for measuring and monitoring PDM.

Prescription End-Date Instruction

This policy, discussed primarily by providers at one MTF who thought that it was a new directive, stipulates that legal prescription use is capped at six months after the date the prescription is issued. A few providers from other MTFs and service branches mentioned vague knowledge of this but were not aware of the exact terms of the limitation; most providers did not mention it at all.

Limitations on Dosages, Pills, and Refills

Several providers across all three service branches reported that prescriptions for *all* controlled substances are capped at a 30-day supply, with refills no sooner than seven days. However, limits vary by provider and MTF, with some providers reporting that standard order sets at some facilities provide a 90-day supply, some noting 30-dose limits for non–chronic pain patients and others reporting 30-day limits for those with chronic pain. Still others reported higher limits, such as 60 days, and more for deployments. One pharmacist said that, although those on controlled substances should not be deployed, this restriction is sometimes waived. A few providers noted that each provider determines prescription and dosage limits on a case-by-case basis. Providers at one medical center recently adjusted the default prescription pill amounts for certain opioids in an attempt to further prevent misuse.

Planned Titration

Few providers said they plan for the eventual titration of patients off of their medications. Some providers expressed concern that lack of such planning could perpetuate misuse because it fails to communicate to patients the expectation that pharmacotherapy is temporary. Two providers reported planning for eventual tapering. Both reported following their own tapering plans rather than any established guidelines. One physician reported that he was starting to receive titration notes from the pain specialist recommending that he titrate some patients off of their pain medications. He said he welcomed the titration note because it gives him the opportunity to work with the specialist to explore alternatives for patients.

Chronic Pain, High-Utilizer, Polypharmacy Data and Risk Stratification

A few providers at two MTFs discussed use of high-intensity user lists (i.e., lists of ADSMs who use services frequently and are prescribed multiple medications) and categorization by level of risk. According to one WTU clinical pharmacist, medical command assigns each ADSM a color that indicates that ADSM's level of risk for PDM. The risk categories are based on the number of prescriptions an ADSM has and service member profiles. The risk color determines the level of medication management needed. Physicians and clinical pharmacists receive these CHUP data and use them to determine the level of medication management needed. Physicians at MTFs that use these data described relying on them (and on the pharmacists) to do the greater part of assessing patients for potential PDM.

Clinical Pharmacy, Case Management, and Interdisciplinary Coordination

A few of the MTFs we visited have clinical pharmacists or nurse case managers who work with individual ADSMs to review all medications, order urine drug screens, and review drug risks and side effects. Providers at facilities with clinical pharmacists tended to rely on them to assess and manage risk for patients on high-risk medications (i.e., those with high potential for abuse or adverse events, such as DEA schedule II narcotics) and to communicate concerns to physicians. Some case managers also reported taking on these duties, although, more frequently, they were involved only in the cases of "complex" patients, including those on multiple medications, those with chronic pain, those with suspected PDM, or those with previous medical or behavioral issues. One case manager described her role this way:

> If I have a chronic pain patient, I monitor [that patient]. I have access to [the patient's] provider notes, so I can see them. Anyone I send to an outside provider, I have [that patient] sign a release and monitor [that patient]. I review [the patient's] notes and [the patient's] progress and will then notify the PCM.

Pharmacy technicians also regularly check the EMR for drug overlaps and send alerts to physicians, but the EMR misses medications purchased outside of TRICARE or prescribed by certain types of providers.[3]

Medication Reconciliation

With a few exceptions, providers did not discuss medical reconciliation as part of standard care. The few providers who mentioned it described it as a process that involves the clinical pharmacist or physician matching the patient's medications—usually self-reported—with the medications listed in the EMR. Reconciliation typically does not involve counting pills unless the service member is at high risk, such as those in the WTU, but is a more general process to ensure that all of the

---

[3] For example, prescriptions written by dentists would not necessarily be captured.

medications the service member is taking are legitimately prescribed and documented and to better understand the patient's history.

Referral for Complementary and Alternative Pain Management
A variety of providers mentioned the value of complementary practices, such as mind/body programs, chiropractic services, acupuncture, meditation, and physical therapy, as well as nonsurgical pain management interventions. However, providers also mentioned the lack of access to these practices either because they are not available within the MTF or because there are long waiting lists both within and outside the MTF. The providers noted that, in most regions, the largest MTF, often a large hospital, provides these services but might have long wait times and limited services and, in some cases, is not located near the MTF. One physician felt that the lack of these resources can dictate a patient's course of treatment: "At [large MTF], they have pain management specialists, acupuncturists, lots of different modalities for treating pain. Here we usually use pharmacy to treat pain." A few providers also reported pursuing certifications in these programs themselves in order to better serve their patients.

Pill Disposal and Take-Back
DEA regulations prohibit pharmacies from taking back controlled substances. Most MTFs participate in planned take-back events, which typically occur on every base twice a year and are reportedly very successful. Providers generally agree that additional take-backs and clearer procedures for disposing of medications would be useful. One provider commented, "I would love to tell my patients to bring them back, but we legally can't take anything."

Awareness of Policies and Clinical Practice Guidelines Aimed at Identifying Prescription Drug Misuse
After we asked providers about policies and procedures for *preventing* PDM, we discussed policies and procedures for *identifying* PDM. Once again, several key themes emerged during our discussion with the providers across the nine MTFs. Here we provide an overview of these

key themes, and the rest of the section provides a detailed discussion of each theme:

- Despite technical and operational barriers, providers reported depending primarily on electronic systems to identify PDM.
  - AHLTA/CHCS was the primary reported mechanism for identifying ADSMs with PDM; there was variation in how the system is used across providers, MTFs, and service branches.
  - Perceived barriers to using EMRs to prevent PDM include an antiquated interface, a lack of interoperability between departments (such as primary care or ER), and limited medication-tracking history.
- State PDMPs could be extremely useful for identifying PDM but were not reported as being used consistently.
  - Providers indicated that there is currently no mechanism other than PDMPs for tracking purchases made outside of TRI-CARE.
  - Perceived barriers to using the system effectively to identify PDM include lack of access by providers who are not licensed, DoD restrictions prohibiting reporting to the state PDMP, and lack of interface between state PDMPs.
- The Military Personnel Drug Abuse Testing Program (MPDATP) is thought to be an effective way to deter and identify PDM, but providers perceive some limitations.
  - Providers regard the MPDATP as a useful deterrent to PDM and as a way to detect misuse.
  - Perceived limitations include the difficulty in determining whether use of a prescription drug, identified through a urine screen, could be defined as clinically indicated use.
- Many providers follow clinic-level procedures or own experiences and clinical judgment to identify PDM.
  - Reported procedures include high-risk medication and SP review, pre-appointment chart review, ER-specific practices, and patient behavioral cues.
  - Providers reported relying on own clinical experiences and judgment to determine the presence of PDM.

Despite Barriers, Providers Depend Primarily on Electronic Medical Records to Identify Prescription Drug Misuse

Most of the providers with whom we spoke, across MTFs and regions, discussed the AHLTA/CHCS as the primary mechanism for identifying patients who might be misusing prescription medications. However, despite recent improvements to this system, most also pointed to substantial barriers, including an antiquated interface, the majority of patient prescription data being embedded "deep within" CHCS and not easily accessible, a lack of interoperability between departments (such as primary care or ER), and limited medication-tracking history. Although AHLTA/CHCS is used at all MTFs, how the MTFs use the system to identify patients with PDM varies. How providers within MTFs use the system, depending on their roles and their specialties (see Table 4.6), also varies. In terms of identifying PDM, most MTFs

Table 4.6
Use of Armed Forces Health Longitudinal Technology Application Composite Health Care System and Other Electronic Medical Records to Identify Prescription Drug Misuse That Our Interviewees Mentioned

Facility	EMR Usage
1	For every patient, the PCM checks AHLTA for recent prescriptions. For patients of concern, such as those with frequent ER visits, the case manager checks the entire history in CHCS. For higher-risk and polypharmacy patients, a clinical pharmacist creates the CHUP list and gives it to the PCM.
2	For patients of concern, the ER physician does a search in AHLTA/CHCS for past orders and a WTU case manager pulls history from AHLTA/CHCS.
3	For patients of concern, the PCM requests prescription information.
4	For patients of concern, a nurse conducts a chart review of the Aeromedical Services Information Management System to look for frequent waivers and cross-references with AHLTA/CHCS. For patients in ADAPT identified with the PCM, ADAPT puts a flag in AHLTA/CHCS. For patients on SP agreements, the PCM puts a flag in AHLTA/CHCS (this is often entered in a medication field).
5	A pain committee reviews a report that includes all controlled substances prescribed in the area to ADSMs and discusses patients of concern. A utilization manager reviews all schedule II prescriptions purchased through TRICARE insurance.

Table 4.6—Continued

Facility	EMR Usage
6	A PCM (or designee) reviews AHLTA/CHCS for care received within or outside DoD facilities and enters the pain contract as a medication flag in CHCS, which acts like a drug interaction to alert providers. A pharmacist runs a report on high utilizers (any patient prescribed more than five controlled substances per month or who have seen three doctors for controlled substances per month) and sends the report to providers every two months.
7	For patients who are frequent fliers (i.e., those who regularly visit the doctor to obtain medication), a PCM (or designee) enters them in AHLTA. For patients of concern, a PCM checks prescription history in AHLTA/CHCS and a pharmacist checks Pharmacy Data Transaction Service data in AHLTA.
8	For patients with drug-seeking behavior, an ER physician puts notes about behavior in AHLTA/CHCS. For patients of concern, an embedded nurse case manager checks CHCS. For all patients, a pharmacist uses the system to check for drug overlaps; pharmacist technicians receive an alert.
9	A pain specialist created a dummy drug (a placeholder medication variable) in CHCS that shows physician contact information and interacts with all the opiates (this was discontinued due to technical difficulties). A pain specialist encourages PCMs to upload SP and pain agreements into the Health Artifact and Image Management Solution (a designated space in AHLTA/CHCS). For patients of concern, an ER clinical social worker checks Pharmacy Data Transaction Service in AHLTA. For all patients, an ER physician uses Centris (the system for hospital inpatients and ER patients) to log prescriptions and CHCS to search prescription histories for patients of concern.

and providers generally use the system to search for recent and past prescriptions and to identify patients who are on an SP or other type of high-risk medication agreement and who might be seeking medications outside of their agreements. Some MTFs also use or cross-reference other EMRs that do not interface with AHLTA/CHCS, such as the Aeromedical Services Information Management System and Centris, an electronic health management system used in one of the emergency rooms, as well as the state prescription drug databases. Table 4.6 highlights some of the ways providers and MTFs use AHLTA/CHCS and other EMRs to identify ADSMs with possible PDM.

Many providers with whom we spoke noted barriers to using EMRs to prevent PDM, which are similar across MTFs and service branches. Barriers that providers mentioned the most frequently include the following:

- *no mechanism for tracking non-TRICARE medication purchases:* Medications purchased outside of TRICARE insurance from civilian pharmacies are not tracked in AHLTA/CHCS.
- *time lag:* If a civilian provider writes a prescription and the patient uses TRICARE insurance to purchase the medication, there is a time lag between when the prescription is written and when it shows up in the system.
- *inconsistent flagging for patients on agreements:* Flags for identifying ADSMs on an SP or other agreement are not used consistently across MTFs and are not always visible in AHLTA/CHCS.
- *lack of flagging for at-risk patients other than those on agreements:* Although there are sometimes flags for patients on SP or other medication agreements, there are no flags for patients thought to be at risk for PDM for other reasons, such as a positive screen for history of PDM that might be conducted in a military drug treatment program (e.g., ADAPT, SARP, ASAP).
- *lack of system interface:* Dental and inpatient or ER EMRs do not typically interface with AHLTA/CHCS, so doctors cannot see all prescriptions.
- *poor AHLTA/CHCS crossover:* Most historical prescription information is "deep within" CHCS. Providers report having to "do a lot of digging" to find prescription histories. Providers also report that the AHLTA medication profile is not always up to date, so they have to look in CHCS, which is much more time-consuming and thus sometimes overlooked.
- *limited tracking time frame:* For medications ordered by outside providers, CHCS goes back only 180 days.

State Prescription Drug Monitoring Programs Are Not Used Consistently

State PDMPs were available in all four states we visited, and some of the providers with whom we spoke at each facility reported using their state's PDMP to check on prescriptions purchased outside of

TRICARE insurance by "members of concern" (i.e., patients with polypharmacy and those with frequent complaints and medication requests). As mentioned previously, there is currently no mechanism other than PDMP for tracking purchases made outside of TRICARE. When we asked providers about the use of PDMP, pharmacists had the greatest familiarity and felt that physicians also regularly access these databases; physicians, on the other hand, reported using the databases infrequently themselves but believed that pharmacists regularly access them for patients of concern. One pharmacist reported that he writes a note in AHLTA after he checks the state PDMP so the physician can access the information.

Perceived barriers to using the system effectively to identify PDM that the providers with whom we spoke mentioned include the lack of access by providers who are not licensed in that particular state to access the PDMP; privacy restrictions prohibiting DoD from reporting to the state PDMP information about ADSM prescriptions purchased through the MHS; and the lack of interface between state PDMPs. One physician noted that the licensing restriction is challenging for military providers who tend to change installations, and thus states, fairly regularly. Providers generally agree that access to and consistent use of the state PDMPs is a critical step in preventing misuse but that the lack of interface between the state and military systems impedes full and accurate assessment. Frequent PCS among ADSMs, as well as the ease with which ADSMs can cross state boundaries to purchase medication outside of TRICARE, creates several loopholes in state-specific tracking systems. Providers suggested that access to a single tracking system to track TRICARE and external to TRICARE purchases within and across multiple states would close some of these loopholes.

The Military Personnel Drug Abuse Testing Program Is Thought to Be Effective

Providers with whom we spoke regard the MPDATP, which requires all ADSMs to undergo random urinalysis drug testing—including pharmaceutical drugs, illegal drugs, and other drugs of abuse—once a year and permits commanders to implement drug testing to detect drug abuse at their discretion, as a useful deterrent and as a way to detect misuse. However, the providers with whom we spoke also observed several limitations with the MPDATP. When a service member tests positive for a prescription drug, the medical review officer typically contacts the provider to determine whether the use of the medication in the service member's drug screen was clinically indicated (i.e., there is an active prescription). The providers with whom we spoke report that, in the past, medical review officers had difficulty determining whether prescriptions identified through the MPDATP were clinically indicated and prescribed because of lack of clear policies (or lack of knowledge about policies) regarding the definition of *clinically indicated use*. Although a 2011 Army regulation limits the length of time ADSMs can use prescribed controlled-substance medications to six months from the date it was dispensed (MEDCOM Regulation 40-51 [Assistant Chief of Staff for Health Policy and Services, 2011]), few providers mentioned this. Two providers noted that the MPDATP urinalyses do not seem to be conducted randomly or annually and that this perception among ADSMs could impede the test's effectiveness as a deterrent to PDM. A pain specialist said that the MPDATP, although testing for many opioids, does not test for a full panel of drugs, which has created a loophole for certain medications, such as tramadol.

Providers can also conduct clinic-level urinalyses for high-risk patients and patients on SP and other medication agreements, although there is wide variation in whether and how often these are used. This risk profile is a compilation of an ADSM's physical and mental health assessments, as well as a review of their behavioral and administrative records. One provider suggested that the provider-level UA panel include more drugs (a panel of 100) and that every ADSM should undergo a full panel at least annually as part of the risk profile.

Many Providers Follow Clinic-Level Procedures or Clinical Judgment

The providers with whom we spoke reported that they follow clinic-specific procedures and, at times, rely on their own experiences and clinical judgment to detect PDM among ADSMs. Procedures were similar across regions and sites but tended to vary by provider type, according to role. For example, according to providers, nurses and case managers are more likely than physicians to review charts prior to visits. Clinic-specific procedures and personal practice principles that providers mentioned include the following:

- *high-risk medication and SP review:* medication record review by nurse case managers of a weekly medical compliance report that includes all prescriptions filled under TRICARE for high-risk patients and for patients on SP agreements
- *pre-appointment schedule and chart review*
  - As nurses review the appointment schedule for the day, they select people in advance who might be problematic because they have multiple prescriptions or frequent visits, and they assign screening tests or coordinate with pain management to understand more about each patient's history.
  - Technicians and nurses "scrub" the provider schedules three days prior to appointments to see what visits will entail. They look at the visit reason and then do appropriate research and preparation. For example, if the patient is coming in for an ER follow-up visit, they access the ER files. If they do not have the patient's discharge information, they request records from the ER or ask patients to bring them.
  - Review the patient history, determine what other providers the patient has seen, and look at whether other issues might correlate with substance misuse, such as frequent visits to orthopedists and behavioral health counselors.
  - If, upon chart review, the nurses find multiple refills out of the ordinary, they call the patient in to talk face to face.
- *ER-specific practices*
  - Assess the nature of the complaint, and, if warranted, check the full prescription history in CHCS.
  - "Put out a page" (on the hospital paging system) for a particular provider or case manager who is familiar with the patient to see that patient; some patients will leave after hearing the page if the patient has a history with that provider.
  - An ER-specific social worker reviews records and meets with patients whom an ER physician suspects of drug-seeking following ER treatment.

- *attention to patient behavioral flags:* Pharmacists and nurses in particular reported paying attention to behavioral cues from patients that could indicate PDM. These cues include patients doing the following:
  - going through full prescriptions in a short time frame and requesting early refills
  - reporting loss of a large amount of medication
  - requesting a specific drug (or citing an allergy to an undesired drug)
  - coming in for a refill on the exact day they are due for renewal
  - showing irritability and visible signs of withdrawal
  - having slurred speech or mentioning that the dosage was not sufficient
  - acting "high" or "weird"
  - displaying illogical prescription patterns
  - consistently trying to see another provider
  - frequently showing up in the ER.

Providers also reported that sometimes the unit commander or ADSMs themselves will report concerns regarding overall functioning.

Of note, many providers reported relying on "a sense" or "gut feeling" to determine the presence of PDM. One nurse stated, "I think [that] the literature shows that docs miss [PDM] roughly half the time. They just have no idea [even] when they think they do."

Managing and Treating Prescription Drug Misuse After Identification

In the last part of the discussion on policies and procedures, we focused on how providers manage and treat PDM after it is identified. Because it is relevant for interpreting the basis of these providers' knowledge of effective treatment, we also discussed the extent to which various types of providers received specific training for managing and treating ADSMs with PDM.

Consistent with our general findings in the previous two sections related to preventing and identifying PDM, the providers with whom we spoke once again identified a variety of steps that might be taken once PDM was identified to manage and treat the problem, and none seemed to be specified as a consistent pathway regardless of provider type or MTF. A variety of factors appeared to influence the pathway.

We also discovered in our discussion with providers across MTFs that training in the treatment of PDM varied quite a bit across provider types and MTFs. Awareness of specific available training was mixed, although several health providers noted the development of local and regional initiatives, which we discuss at the end of this section.

Steps Taken After Prescription Drug Misuse Is Identified Vary and Might Depend on Multiple Factors

Although providers did not refer to specific DoD instructions, policies, or CPGs, they reported being aware of the following possible pathways for ADSMs once PDM is identified: (1) medical, (2) behavioral health and substance abuse treatment, and (3) administrative.

According to providers, the medical pathway could include a provider titrating the member off the medication; putting the member on an SP or other agreement if the member is not already on one; assigning the member a new provider; referring the member to a pain specialist (if they have not seen one already) and complementary therapies or detoxing them through the MTF or referring them to a civilian medical detoxification facility. The behavioral health and substance use treatment pathway might involve referral to a mental health therapist, a military substance abuse treatment program, or a civilian treatment program. The administrative pathway, as providers perceive it, involves notifying the service member's unit commander and, potentially, a medical evaluation board review followed by administrative separation from the military.

Pathways are not mutually exclusive and might vary according a range of factors, including how the PDM is identified; the providers' personal beliefs about how PDM should be managed and treated; any existing protocols and whether providers adhere to them; the availability of appropriate alternatives to medication; provider and commander opinions about the service member's circumstances and potential to recover; and the level of adherence (by commanders, MTFs, and service) to what providers frequently call the military's zero tolerance policy for drug abuse. In this section, we describe what we learned about each of the three pathways.

Medical Pathway

When medical providers identify PDM, rather than having PDM identified through a positive MPDATP urine drug screen, they take a variety of steps that depend on the extent of the PDM, patient history, and the provider's clinical judgment. In some cases, physicians titrate the patient off the medication and seek alternatives for the patient, including referring the patient to pain management for nonsurgical procedures and for complementary practices, such as chiropractic or acupuncture, either on or off the base. Pain specialists reported that they either manage the titration themselves or send them back to the PCM for titration. Although most providers discussed SP and other agreements as mechanisms for preventing misuse for patients on opioid therapy for chronic pain or long-term opioid-replacement therapy for opioid addiction (e.g., use of Suboxone or methadone), with violation of the agreement possibly indicating PDM, some providers also mentioned the agreements as a way to closely monitor ADSMs who are starting to exhibit signs of PDM.

In cases of more-severe dependence, several physicians from a variety of MTFs said they refer the patient to an offsite, inpatient detoxification facility, while a couple of providers said they provide medical detox to the patient themselves. Several providers noted a lack of detoxification resources within MHS for patients with dependence. As one physician stated, "If an extensive detox is recommended, we have nowhere to send them. We sent one guy to [an off-site civilian facility more than 1,000 miles from the base]." Another physician, noting the potential administrative consequences from a formal referral to a detoxification facility, described his approach this way: "I know I can detox them myself and no one else is involved, which is better for their careers. It's not optimal."

With a few exceptions, evidence-based pharmacological maintenance, tapering, and anticraving medications for opiate dependence (e.g., buprenorphine with naloxone, oral or injectable naltrexone) are not typically used within any MTF we visited. Further, providers seem confused about whether these treatments are allowable within the MHS as a whole or by specific service branch. Some providers reported using buprenorphine with naloxone (trade name Suboxone) to treat "pain but not addiction," and some reported that some ADSMs receive Suboxone from civilian providers to facilitate tapering. Physicians' reasons for not using Suboxone to treat addiction included the provider not knowing military regulations regarding the medication; not having the DEA "x-waiver" needed to specifically treat addiction (versus pain only); not wanting to be flooded with requests for Suboxone; and, in some cases, not subscribing to treating opioid addiction with an opioid. There was not much mention of naltrexone, although one substance abuse counselor noted receiving a few inquiries about it, but mostly for alcohol dependence, not opioid dependence.

Behavioral Health and Substance Abuse Treatment Pathway

In addition to, or in lieu of, medical intervention, many medical providers also refer patients who exhibit PDM to a pain psychologist, pain management support group, mind/body program, mental health specialist, or military SUD treatment facility (e.g., ADAPT, SARP, ASAP). If the patient is referred to behavioral health, either mental health or SUD treatment, behavioral medicine might handle the medical aspects of titration, but this seems to vary by MTF and provider. Some medical providers refer patients to a mental health specialist if there is one embedded in the medical practice or discuss the patient with a pain committee or other interdisciplinary group, while others refer the patient directly to the military SUD treatment program. Navy providers in particular noted that ADSMs are sometimes referred to drug and alcohol program advisers, who are embedded in units and responsible for informing ADSMs of available treatment options.

Although most, but not all, providers are aware of the option of referring a patient directly to an SUD treatment program for further assessment (per DoDD 1010.4), many providers mentioned several impediments to doing so, including not having leverage to get the service member to go without notifying the member's commander, perceived administrative ramifications to the service member if they do notify the commander, and fear of violating patient confidentiality.

Although some providers refer the patient directly to an SUD treatment program, many providers encourage patients to self-refer, which they believe will allow them to circumvent any administrative consequences and will spare them from commander notification. If an ADSM tests positive for illicit use of a prescription drug (i.e., the member did not have a prescription or the prescription is older than six months) on the MPDATP, the unit commander (according to providers) is required to make a referral to a substance use treatment program for further assessment. Because of the chain of command involved in the custody of the MPDATP urinalysis results, providers believe that referral of ADSMs with PDM to SUD treatment programs comes from commanders more frequently than from physicians.

Administrative Pathway

Provider perspectives on administrative processes for PDM vary, with some of the providers with whom we spoke interpreting the DoD instruction for illicit-drug use and PDM as identical and rigid, with administrative separation imminent regardless of treatment (i.e., they perceive a strict zero tolerance policy and are not aware of exceptions for PDM), while others note extreme variability in administrative outcomes that depend on a variety of patient-, provider- and command-level factors. A nurse case manager explained her perception of the regulations this way:

> Firstly, there's zero tolerance for drugs in the military. If the person is active duty and comes in and lets you know [the person has] a problem, a lot of times, they're very good about getting treatment. A person [who] normally comes forward like that will be sent through treatment, but there's still a zero tolerance policy. If we catch [use] on a drug screen, and [the person tests] positive for a prescription opiate for which [the person does not] have a prescription, [the person is] discharged immediately.

However, an ADAPT counselor viewed it somewhat differently:

> In terms of an administrative separation, it depends on the situation. There's supposed to be a DoD policy surrounding zero toler-

ance but . . . like everything in the military, it's commander discretion. Recently, it's been "if it's your second incidence, you have to go." We treat patients before their discharge, but it's ultimately under command's discretion. The commander can pull a patient out of the facility and kick [that person] out of the military. Our program is between six months to a year, and you are undeployable [during that time]. If you are undeployable for a year then you theoretically should get [a medical evaluation board review, during which an ADSM's "fitness for deployment" is assessed, frequently resulting in administrative separation from the military].

Differing provider perspectives of the administrative consequences of PDM might affect whether ADSMs with PDM are referred for treatment and, perhaps paradoxically, how they are viewed within the military if they are referred. Providers might be reluctant to refer members to receive the services they need to help them manage their PDM because they fear administrative consequences and stigma for ADSMs that are equivalent to those for illicit-drug use, even if the ADSMs self-refer to treatment. SUD counselors widely acknowledged the stigma that accompanies any type of ADSM visit to their departments (across SARP, ADAPT, and ASAP) and said that service members, perhaps understandably, are reluctant to seek help even when they recognize the need for it.

Military Substance Use Disorder Treatment Programs Might Not Be Appropriate for All Prescription Drug Misuse

Some medical providers with whom we spoke believe that PDM develops from a clinically appropriate prescription and chronic pain does not necessarily warrant formal SUD treatment or the perceived potential administrative consequences that treatment referral triggers. Moreover, because some of the military substance abuse treatment programs treat primarily alcohol abuse and dependence, these programs might not be prepared to treat PDM, particularly PDM that develops because of ongoing chronic pain. Further, some of the medical providers with whom we spoke believe that traditional substance abuse treatment might not be appropriate for some types of PDM. One pain specialist put it this way: "I think *addiction* and *dependence* here are used interchangeably when they shouldn't be. This blurs the lines between valid appropriate treatment and inappropriate treatments." As noted by an ADAPT provider,

> Our current mechanism for treatment wouldn't be very effective for someone who isn't necessarily abusing drugs but becoming more physiologically dependent on [them]. Our current true treatment and after care (six to 12 months of bimonthly meetings) [are] focused on alcohol abuse or dependence. We will bring people who are diagnosed with a drug-related dependence diagnosis, and we can work them in there. Generally, those people are ones [who] specifically abused [prescription drugs].

A clinical social worker described SARP this way:

> SARP does not provide prescription drug abuse treatment per se. [It is] focused specifically on alcohol and illegal drug use. [It does not] focus on those patients with a real need for these medications. There's one place in this area that works specifically and only with prescription drug use; if the command is willing to pay for it, then we can send people there.

Mandatory Prescription Drug Misuse Training, Regional and Local Training Initiatives, and Participation Barriers

Following our discussion of policies and procedures, we asked providers about any training they had received on PDM either within or outside of the military, about regional and local training initiatives, and about barriers to providers receiving training. Although some providers recalled having PDM training during their medical or nursing certification processes, several said they had not had, and were not aware of, any subsequent training through the military. Others noted participation in an online Swank HealthCare training related to PDM. Several pharmacists also noted administrative (e.g., MEDCOM, the Navy Bureau of Medicine and Surgery) policies that explain polypharmacy policies that touch on PDM. Despite the growing availability of training, particularly online training not necessarily focused on military providers, participation in training seems to differ across MTFs (see

Table 4.7). In fact, some providers reported insufficient, inadequate, or no training at all related to PDM.

Awareness, accessibility, and prioritization of PDM might play a role in the varied use of these resources. One family practice nurse noted that an NP with whom she works admitted to having insuf-

Table 4.7
Variations in Training Type Across Medical Treatment Facilities

Facility	Type of Training and Local or Regional Initiative Reported	Overall Provider Sentiment About Training
1	Project ECHO VTC; module on polypharmacy; lectures from pharmacist and addictionologist, continuing medical education, and SP program orientation; internal meetings and journal club	ECHO VTC is good, but timing makes attendance difficult, and it is open only to certain staff. There is little to no training other than continuing-education units; training is needed on prescribing opiates and identifying PDM.
2	Informal annual training on medication reconciliation procedures; guest lectures from addictionologist and pain specialist	There is no training specifically focused on identifying and treating PDM.
3	Weekly telehealth VTC with large MTF in the region (focus more on pain management than PDM, but discussion includes identification of PDM)	Provider education is needed on prescribing opioids.
4	Monthly professional staff meetings; informal presentations on prescriptions	No comments on training needs
5	Annual mandatory training on prescribing high-risk medications; annual training on pain management; pro-staff meeting to discuss pain management	More training is needed not only on prescribing practices for providers but also for commanders and supervisors.
6	Annual computer-based training on prescription and illicit drugs, Swank (computer-based) training; computer-based training training on PDM	More provider training is needed on prescribing practices and setting realistic expectations for patients with chronic pain.
7	Swank training on PDM that includes video scenarios and best practices	More provider education is needed on prescribing practices and alternatives to prescription medication; pharmacy education

Table 4.7—Continued

Facility	Type of Training and Local or Regional Initiative Reported	Overall Provider Sentiment About Training
8	ECHO VTC (just starting); pain management class for nurses, social workers, doctors; Lean Six Sigma project for providers on detecting doctor-shopping; informal interdisciplinary coordination and education	Expand training in alternative pain treatment modalities.
9	ECHO VTC; U.S. Food and Drug Administration–recommended national Risk Evaluation and Mitigation Strategy program for prescribers of high-risk (per Food and Drug Administration definition) medication; service-specific chronic opioid therapy safety program	Educate providers on prescribing guidelines, universal safeguards for patients on chronic opioid therapy, and the nuances of addiction.

NOTE: ECHO = Extension for Community Healthcare Outcomes. VTC = video teleconference.

ficient training and not knowing how to prescribe opiates for people at risk of PDM. Midlevel providers in the sample felt underprepared both to detect and to treat PDM across MTF facilities, including the ER and outpatient clinics, with little in the way of training options. For those aware of training options, the chief obstacle is time. With competing interests, a full patient panel, and substantial administrative duties, several providers cited time as the limiting factor, leading many providers to have only a vague recollection of the training. Despite varied levels of availability and participation, many providers across sites noted that more training is needed on PDM, best prescribing practices, and managing patients on chronic opioid therapy.

Several providers with whom we spoke noted the development of local and regional initiatives to address pain management through training. Larger MTFs seem to be driving the development of new training and opportunities. These initiatives include MTF-wide, interdisciplinary case discussions and Project ECHO VTCs. Interdisciplinary case conferences typically bring together all providers involved with a patient's care, including pain specialists, to establish patient monitoring and care management plans for a specific patient. ECHO VTCs are regarded as excellent training opportunities, with one pain clinic physician noting that "ECHO is also trying to do education pieces with the primary care clinics [to] teach how to prescribe medication," and another commenting, "so we teleconference and become educated [because] we can present our toughest cases."

Larger MTFs also appear to be driving the development of opioid instructional guidelines to support provider education. One physician described his involvement in the development of a pain management and chronic opioid therapy curriculum for physicians and midlevel providers, both within and outside of the MTF. The curriculum has monitoring and evaluation components, informational materials, and provider tools to track and manage care for chronic pain patients. As part of this initiative, physicians are reaching out to providers in the community who provide chronic pain services in an effort to bridge the gap in care continuity for ADSMs. These physicians conduct lectures and briefings on best prescribing practices and management of patients on chronic opiates.[4] As part of the effort to take the project to scale, physicians also have become involved with county advisory personnel.

Perceived Challenges to and Recommendations for Effectively Managing Prescription Drug Misuse

Throughout the interviews, providers who agreed to be interviewed noted a variety of challenges to effectively preventing, identifying, and treating PDM among ADSMs. In this chapter, we summarize key themes that emerged from these conversations regarding the challenges providers faced, as well as their recommendations for more effectively managing and treating ADSMs with PDM; some of the challenges led naturally to a description of how they might be overcome. Toward the end of this chapter, we list other recommendations, made outside of specific challenges faced.

---

[4] A patient can be on a chronic opioid in one of two ways: (1) being a patient with chronic pain who receives opioids as a way of living with the chronic pain (i.e., chronic use) or (2) using opioid-replacement therapy, in which a less psychoactive opioid, such as buprenorphine, Suboxone, or methadone replaces the opioid to which the patient is addicted.

Electronic Health and Monitoring Systems

Providers noted that the current military EMR systems—primarily AHLTA/CHCS and other systems, such as Centris—are fragmented; do not consistently display flags and prescription histories for patients prescribed opioids; are not used the same way across MTFs and other military clinics; and do not, in a standardized, consistent, or visible way, indicate which ADSMs are on SP or other agreements. Many providers believe that enhancing the capacity and use of electronic systems is necessary to effectively prevent and identify PDM and made specific recommendations for doing so. As noted by one physician,

> We also need one computer system for everything. We're on four different systems in the same building. If you had one system, it would be much easier to tell what's going on. I think that would catch a fair amount of errors and misuse.

Providers also described the difficulties inherent to tracking prescriptions purchased outside of TRICARE and noted that more-consistent use of state PDMPs would help remedy this large loophole. Finally, some providers expressed frustration with not being able to upload prescription purchases of military personnel to the state PDMP because different states have different policies regarding who is allowed or required to report in state PDMPs, and some require a license in that state. Others expressed the need for a single, federal system that could track all prescriptions, both within and outside of the MHS, in order to effectively identify PDM.

Specific provider recommendations related to improving electronic records are as follows:

- Create AHLTA icons or flags for (1) ADSMs currently on opioids; (2) ADSMs who have received opioid therapy in the past; (3) ADSMs on SP or other agreements; and (4) ADSMs with medication adherence issues.
- Display in AHLTA the 12-month (instead of six-month) prescription history.
- Monitor all prescriptions, including those purchased out of pocket (without TRICARE) from civilian pharmacies.

- Work with state PDMPs to increase access for military health providers who might not be licensed in the state.
- Upload service member prescription purchases to state PDMPs.
- Create a federal PDMP.

Training and Decision Support

The lack of a well-specified medical approach for detecting, managing, and treating ADSMs with PDM across MTFs, military clinics, service branches, and regions is a clear barrier for effective and consistent management and treatment of these patients. Although providers acknowledge that mandatory training is burdensome and sometimes unmemorable, many think that mandatory training on PDM for PCP in particular is critical to improving the management of PDM. As one physician put it,

> I am hesitant to say we need more training because time is already limited, but it would be valuable to have some training about prescription drug misuse because it's a fairly untouched issue and people have been "winging it" with regard to sole-provider programs, narcotics prescribing, and coordinating the resources within institutions.

A clinical pharmacist thought that every primary care provider should be offered a full day of training conducted by a specialist so the training would stand out from other, computer-based training. Others think that all prescribers and staff who might encounter PDM should receive training.

Providers suggested the following training topics:

- how to recognize PDM
- understanding addiction, tolerance, and dependency
- best practices for prescribing opioids
- CPGs and SP and other agreements
- existing DoD policies around PDM and chronic pain
- universal care methods for pain assessment and pain management.

Providers also recommended ongoing decision support to facilitate prescribing for and management of ADSMs on opioid therapy for chronic pain. A pharmacist noted that decision-support systems for providers could be built into the health care process in addition to training. Along the same lines, an ADAPT specialist suggested that ongoing live meetings would provide sustained decision support and relevant training for providers as they encounter PDM. A nurse case manager suggested expanding ECHO VTC programs.

Patient Education and Self-Management

As mentioned in previously in this chapter, many providers believe that the vast majority of ADSMs who misuse prescription medications do so after first having a clinically indicated medical need for the medications. They therefore misuse them or become addicted accidentally, because they lack knowledge about the risks of the prescription medications they take, how to take them, or the consequences of taking them other than in the manner prescribed. Several providers recommend improving patient education about their pain, prescriptions, and treatment plans, so as to possibly prevent some of the accidental misuse that occurs. They also recommend teaching patients self-management skills to help prevent PDM in the future. Specific recommendations include

- having PCMs or pharmacists educate patients on what to expect from chronic pain and to convey to patients that they might have pain in spite of taking their medication
- providing each patient with a clear road map that outlines the course of treatment so that the patient does not expect to be on medication indefinitely
- improving patient (service member) education about the risk of dependence for the medications the patient is taking if the patient takes them for different durations of time
- teaching patients coping skills to better manage their pain and comorbid psychological issues.

Providers noted that spending additional time with patients is often not feasible in busy clinics that allow for only 15 to 20 minutes with each patient and recommended integrating case managers and clinical pharmacists into these practices to facilitate the additional but much-needed work.

Access to Specialty Pain Management and Complementary Practices

Although some MTFs we visited had pain management clinics and complementary practices, most did not. Providers at MTFs with specialty clinics and with pain specialists noted the tremendous value of these services and specialists in providing appropriate care to ADSMs with chronic pain and alternatives to medication and called for a "well-staffed, interdisciplinary pain management center that provide soldiers with a greater breadth of treatment modalities." Many providers noted the need for a biopsychosocial approach to pain management with ADSMs, who often have complex medical and psychological needs. Another recommendation was to have designated disease managers for chronic pain patients stationed within patient-centered medical homes (PCMHs) and to develop a special patient registry for population-based care of these patients.

Interdisciplinary Coordination

Although some providers described improved interdisciplinary coordination within their settings for patients at risk of or identified with PDM, with regular pain committee meetings occurring among physicians, commanders, pharmacists, and case managers, others noted the lack of coordination in their settings as a real barrier to managing PDM and recommended it as a useful strategy going forward. A major reason for the lack of coordination was a lack of staff, time, and resources needed to coordinate care.

A variety of different tools could be used to try to promote better coordination, one of which has already been mentioned (i.e., more-integrated EMRs). Another tool, assuming that resources are not a significant constraint, is embedding case managers and clinical pharmacists into clinics as dedicated case managers for these problems. One provider specifically recommended having a case manager on site who could fully coordinate care for patients at risk of PDM or with PDM and communicate with other providers, as well as commanders. Assuming that resources for new staff are a constraint, one pain specialist offered yet another recommendation: having pain specialists and primary care work more closely together in those locations where both exist to identify, manage, and treat PDM. Doing so would help reduce the "cultural divide" between pain management and primary care.

Adherence to Guidelines and Policies

Although providers were generally aware of CPGs and MTF, service-specific, and DoD-level policies pertaining to chronic pain and PDM, a fair number were not completely familiar with them. Some observed that policies and practices differed across MTFs, as well as within clinics within the same MTF, while some noted that there was poor adherence with little consequence to providers, and others expressed the need for new guidelines and policies. Providers suggested that, to the extent possible, practices around PDM need to be standardized at least across MTFs and ideally across services, including VA. According to providers, standardization and adherence would close loopholes and, in doing so, increase providers' ability to prevent, identify, and treat PDM. Specific recommendations that were offered to improve knowledge, standardization, and adherence to guidelines and policies were the following:

- Institute programs that increase knowledge of and adherence to CPGs for opioids, including explaining how long people should stay on opioids.
- Develop new guidelines around PDM at the DoD level, rather than the MTF level, with input from a variety of physicians across services, and then facilitate implementation of the new guidelines in primary care clinics.
- Require all providers to use a standardized SP agreement for all patients on chronic opioid therapy, and increase monitoring and enforcement.
- Use standardized screening assessments for all patients who are starting opioid therapy to determine risk for PDM, and provide clear guidelines for how to interpret and apply assessment data.
- Monitor patients on opioid therapy more closely, with 100-panel UAs more than once or twice a year.

- Develop definitive guidelines for treating patients with chronic pain to help providers become more comfortable relying on alternatives and to ensure that patients do not come to expect opioids.
- Incorporate PDM- and pain management–specific curricula and treatment into outpatient SUD treatment, through ADAPT, SARP, and ASAP.
- Clarify administrative policies and procedures for ADSMs identified with PDM, and consider "decriminalizing" PDM to reduce stigma and punitive measures for patients with iatrogenic dependence.
- Standardize ER practices around providing prescriptions for patients with chronic pain; this could help close the ER loophole for prescription drug seekers and limit patient complaints about not being able to get medications in the ER.
- Create standardized metrics for measuring and tracking PDM, and make transparent the number of service member overdose deaths, arrests for diversion, and any other data pertaining to PDM.

Although they do not make up a representative sample of medical providers from across all service branches, medical areas of expertise, or geographic regions of the country, the 66 providers who participated in interviews from the nine MTFs we visited offered numerous ground-floor insights regarding the nature and extent of the PDM problem among ADSMs and offered input on the elements of existing procedures and policies that are currently in place to effectively manage the problem. Numerous themes emerged from these interviewed, despite it being a relatively small sample, including the inconsistent implementation of existing guidelines and policies across MTFs and the need for clearer DoD-wide guidelines given that so many MTFs treat ADSMs from different services. In the Chapter Five, we organize several of the central themes into some recommendations and policy implications based on the additional insights we obtained from our broader literature review.

Recommendations and Conclusions

With more than 52 million Americans—20 percent of the household population[1]—currently reporting the nonmedical use of prescription medication, PDM has become a major problem in the United States (SAMHSA, 2014). PDM imposes serious health risks, including the potential for death from overdose. Indeed, among active-duty personnel, deaths from drug overdoses more than doubled between 2006 and 2011, and 68 percent of these deaths involved prescription medications (Headquarters, Department of the Army, 2012a).

For the military, PDM generates more than just health risks; it also influences combat readiness. The extent of the problem in terms of combat readiness could be substantial. In a recent study of military combat veterans, two-thirds of the veterans identified as prescription opioid misusers self-reported misuse of these prescription opioids while on deployment (Golub and Bennett, 2013). Evidence from TRICARE pharmacy data would suggest that this estimate from a nonrandom sample of combat veterans might not be too far off, given that just over one-quarter of ADSMs received at least one prescription opioid in fiscal year 2010 (Jeffery, May, et al., 2014). Thus, the threat to readiness is real and matters not just for individual service members but also for the entire teams or units to which those service members belong.

The purpose of this report was to provide information to the Office of the Under Secretary of Defense for Personnel and Readiness that could assist in the identification, prevention, and treatment

---

[1] *Household population* is a way of referring to the U.S. general population living in households (as opposed to living in, for example, transitional housing, jails, prisons, or dormitories).

of PDM among active-duty service members. We pursued three different research strategies to assist us in accomplishing this task, and each provided important insights. Our review of the literature helped us understand that little guidance was available in either military policies or civilian clinical guidelines for the management and treatment of PDM. Instead, most of the 20 DoD military policies and clinical guidelines addressing PDM focus on how to define the behavior and the steps to take following identification, not the treatment options or the management of treatment. The same was true for non-DoD and civilian guidelines, however. And very few studies have evaluated prevention and treatment strategies specifically for PDM in either a civilian or military setting. The majority of current guidelines, consensus statements, and published literature focus on heroin abuse, rather than prescription misuse, and note a general lack of evidence of many of the approaches commonly used in practice to predict misuse.

In light of the lack of formal guidance and the lack of evidence base, it was not surprising to learn from the qualitative interviews that providers often rely on their own experience and clinical judgment to detect PDM among ADSMs rather than utilize standard procedures. Although there is some knowledge of CPG for chronic pain, as well as DoD policies around substance abuse and PDM, practices and adherence tend to vary by provider and MTF, with providers noting the need for more-consistent guidelines and greater adherence. The practices employed tended to be clinic-specific rather than military-wide and seemed to vary systematically by provider type, suggesting that the procedures and practices were tied more to general provider approach than to something unique and specific to the PDM problem.

Many providers with whom we spoke called for a more standardized approach to identifying, managing, and treating PDM given the inconsistency across MTFs and clinics. However, without a strong evidence base, it is not possible to definitively say which standardized approach the military should take. Given that implementing a standardized approach is costly, it seems unwise for us to move forward with a recommendation to adopt a standardized approach when we cannot say definitively what that approach should be.

Similarly, nearly all the providers with whom we spoke stated that they relied on existing EMRs as their primary tool to help identify PDM in patients, despite these systems being clunky and inadequate for this purpose. Moreover, many providers suggested that EMRs might be an effective way to better coordinate care of patients with PDM, especially those receiving care across multiple settings or multiple geographic locations. Although many of the providers' recommendations seem worthy of consideration in principle, how to implement them is not clear given the enormous complexity of the DoD's electronic health record system and the myriad of groups that are responsible for pieces of it. Further consideration of how to use the EMR system and how it is evolving in response to other system changes seems to be important before making strong recommendations as to how they can be used to help with the PDM problem.

A common theme in talking with providers that is consistent with our broader literature review is that *the vast majority of people who are diagnosed as having a PDM had medically indicated use before they started misusing the drug.* However, we cannot know, based on existing information, the extent to which this perception is true, particularly given that nonmedical use of any substance is taken very seriously in the military and hence unlikely to be reported. Effective policy that will reduce PDM among ADSMs depends on the key source driving this problem: whether PDM stems from serious medical conditions (in which case policies should be geared toward the health system) or deviant and inappropriate behavior (in which case policies should be geared toward the personnel system).

To assist the military in its effort to better understand the extent to which PDM stems from a medical health issue rather than simple deviant or inappropriate behavior, we developed a compartmental model, described in Chapter Three and presented in Appendix B, that can be parameterized using data available within the military. This analytical tool, once informed by actual data, can provide policymakers with useful information on the extent to which particular avenues generate a greater share of the misuse problem within the military and how well effective identification and diversion to treatment within the medical setting might help reduce the impact of PDM. Based on our understanding from the literature and interviews, it appears that a good share of the problem is indeed generated from medically indicated use, but the analytic tool we outline in this report will be capable of assessing this empirically and determining which behaviors or transitions are driving the bulk of the misuse problem. This sort of information will be useful for deciding how to best target limited prevention and treatment resources.

But what exactly should be done to address the problem of PDM in the military? That answer will depend to some degree on what is found from the analytic tool regarding the share of the problem that misuse among those with a medical indication causes versus misuse among those who are using nonmedically. Informed by insights gleaned from our literature review and interviews with providers, we offer options for consideration that we describe in the rest of this chapter.

Implement and Parameterize the Compartmental Model Developed in This Report to Enable a Clear Assessment of the Extent to Which the Current Prescription Drug Misuse Problem Within the Military Stems from Abuse Following Legitimate Medical Need or Simple Inappropriate Use

Once the model has been parameterized and tested, military leadership can use it to track the evolution of the PDM problem over time (based on trends in key characteristics driving the problem over time), as well as identify the extent to which particular policy approaches (e.g., harsh penalties targeting misusers, or broader implementation of step-down therapies and pain management techniques for patients suffering from a severe injuries causing pain) might be effective at addressing the unique PDM problem that the military faces.

Dedicate Resources to Providing Remedial Training and Support to All Military Health Care Providers in Identifying and Treating Substance Abuse in Patients

Our findings provide strong justification for clinical training of all new and existing medical personnel on identifying and treating addictions (i.e., a comprehensive course providing information on identifying early signs of all addictive behaviors, not just those most problematic today). In doing so, the military can address the current PDM problem and educate its providers on how to identify future potential health problems, such as problems with benzodiazepines, alcohol, or even e-cigarettes. However, the military needs to do more than just provide training. In particular, it needs to make sure that the training that is provided is indeed scientifically supported and effective. It needs to make sure that the material is easy for providers to access and use, giving providers examples of how to identify patients who are at risk for a variety of substances of abuse through the use of a standardized, evidence-based screening tool. Moreover, it needs to educate providers on what to do with patients when they have been screened positive using these tools, linking them to the most effective care.

In addition to training providers, however, the military needs to be aware of and address for providers the system- and patient-level barriers that make providing linked care so difficult to achieve. Removal of patient barriers could be achieved through the broad-scale implementation of a modified-limited use policy, such as the Army's Confidential Alcohol Treatment and Education Program (CATEP), but applied to PDM. Health system barriers might be overcome through electronic connectivity between providers, brief case-management strategies, and supportive care activities to better connect care received in the medical and specialty treatment settings (Cucciare and Timko, 2015; Molfenter et al., 2012; Rapp et al., 2008). These are just a couple of strategies currently being adopted within the civilian health care system in light of mandates associated with the Affordable Care Act to better integrate behavioral and medical health care for people suffering from SUDs (Humphreys and Frank, 2014; Ghitza and Tai, 2014).

Facilitate Interdisciplinary Provider Coordination in Approaches to Identifying and Treating Prescription Drug Misuse, as Well as the Transition to Integrated Care

Changes in civilian and military health care systems that include care coordination through PCMHs provide a natural opportunity for expanded prevention, identification, and treatment of PDM. Several models of PCMH are currently being implemented within the military sector (Nathan, 2013). In MTFs that have already begun to make these changes, providers reported greater collaboration through the use of embedded case managers and behavioral health therapists to facilitate chart reviews and communication about and manage ADSMs with PDM. Given that service integration is relatively new, it is important to continue to monitor these efforts to help inform how to best design these systems for the future.

For Those Suffering with Chronic Pain, Expand the Availability of and Access to Pain Management and Patient-Centered Practices Within the Military Health System

It was clear from our discussion with providers that pain management and patient-centered, complementary services are not readily available or accessible to those suffering from chronic pain. Providers believe that these practices can support treatment for patients with chronic pain but that few within the MHS provide these services, and, where they are available, waiting lists can be long. Treatment outside of the MHS is also possible, but coverage for that care might be limited, and the tracking of these alternative treatments is often difficult.

It was also clear, however, that providers were uncertain about which strategies or guidelines to follow at the different facilities. In light of this, and given the challenges of managing PDM patients suffering from either acute or chronic pain, the military could benefit from the development of remedial training for all new military health care providers on this topic as well. This is not a content area generally included in civilian training systems, and yet it is a comorbid condition frequently encountered within the military in particular. This training, which could commence before the medical and paramedical personnel are first assigned to their posts, would provide the military the opportunity to educate its medical providers on how to use a single standardized assessment tool for identifying pain patients at risk of a variety of substances of misuse (e.g., prescription opioids, alcohol, benzodiazepines) and what to do when ADSMs are identified positive (i.e., at risk). Clear directives could be provided to all medical and paramedical personnel on the policies, protocols, and clinical guidelines that the military believes are the most effective to follow for patients in these circumstances, as well as provide clear directives to providers regarding the role of pharmacotherapies for treating opioid (or even alcohol) misuse.

Encourage the Use of State Prescription Drug Monitoring Programs

Enhanced policies and procedures to direct military providers to state PDMPs to check for purchases made outside of the TRICARE system would help reduce risk of overprescribing. Potential challenges to this approach include making sure that someone at each military medical facility or clinic has access to the state's PDMP (different states have different rules regarding who is allowed to access their PDMPs). Potential policy changes might be needed to fully realize the benefit, such as allowing military health providers access to state PDMPs or requiring prescriptions purchased through TRICARE to be included in state PDMPs. Nonetheless, such changes in policies pertaining to access to existing state PDMPs are likely to happen more expeditiously than the adoption of the military's own PDMP, which, in many ways, would be even more effective, particularly if it would link to state PDMPs. However, broad-scale development of a military PDMP that can link to state PDMPs is considerably more costly to design and implement than a stand-alone military PDMP would be.

Determine Whether Military Substance Abuse Programs Should Provide Unique Treatment for Service Members Who Develop Dependence on Prescription Medications

The military should explore the potential use of pharmacological maintenance, tapering, and anticraving medications for opiate dependence (e.g., buprenorphine with naloxone or oral, injectable, or extended-release naltrexone). These treatments have been shown to be potentially effective for opioid-dependent populations and might prove viable treatment options for the unique military population. Although there are administrative and practical complexities to providing pharmacological treatments for substance abuse and dependence to ADSMs, adoption of these pharmacotherapies could facilitate and expedite recovery and reintegration of service members into active duty. Other evidence-based behavioral therapies tailored for people with PDM, including those suffering from opioid misuse and chronic pain, also exist. However, all of these options involve costs (time to modify policies so as to allow pharmacotherapies for PDM, resources to set up specialized behavioral therapies for patients suffering from chronic pain, education of clinicians regarding how to taper patients off of addictive prescription drugs, and monitoring systems to watch patients as they are tapered down).

If the number of ADSMs who seek or receive treatment for PDM remains fairly small, broad adoption of any of these approaches will unlikely be cost-effective. Thus, it is important to first identify the size of the unmet need among ADSMs with PDM, which might be done using a tool such as that on which we report here. Once the size of this hidden population is known, one must consider the unique characteristics of these patients (e.g., comorbid conditions that are most common or whether nonmedical use is more common). With that information, it will be possible to then consider whether any or all of the available treatment options for opioid dependence might be considered. If the analysis tool suggests that PDM will continue to grow within the military because of prolonged military engagements, attention to building and sustaining the internal treatment capacity will definitely be needed.

Consider Adoption, Implementation, and Improved Dissemination of a U.S. Department of Defense–Wide Limited-Use Policy

DoD policies toward substance abuse are quite complex but generally emphasize a zero tolerance approach to controlled-substance use, including the nonmedical use of a prescription drug. CATEP offers an alternative model for managing PDM. CATEP was designed with the explicit purpose of encouraging ADSMs to self-refer to treatment for alcohol problems before something severe happened. It encourages soldiers to self-refer by allowing them to do so without commander notification and hence without risk of separation from the Army. In fact, the Army's policy explicitly states that soldiers can self-refer to treatment and still be promoted, even while receiving treatment.

Similar limited-use policies specific to PDM exist today in the Army (AR 600-85, 2012 [Headquarters, Department of the Army, 2012b], p. 25, 4-2) and Navy (OPNAVINST 5350.4D, , 2009 [Director, Personal Readiness and Community Support Branch, 2009], enc. 2, § e, p. 12), although they vary in terms of allowable behaviors and possible administrative actions. These policies are buried in documents that are quite complex, and the documents overall send a strong message of zero tolerance for these behaviors. Hence it is not surprising that we found very few military medical providers from these services who were even aware of the ability to self-refer to treatment for PDM. Those who were aware retained their belief that the risk of disposition from the military was a strong deterrent to ADSMs actually doing a self-referral.

Our reading of these policies suggests that expansion of existing limited-use policies, such as those in the Navy or Army, for PDM might be desirable as a DoD-wide policy. Doing so would eliminate confusion that the services' taking different approaches causes and help providers develop strategies on how they might be able to intervene when they encounter ADSMs with such problems. However, it was beyond the scope of the current effort to do a full legal review of these policies, so we acknowledge that such a review is necessary before a formal recommendation of a DoD-wide policy could be made.

At the very least, broader awareness of the policies that already exist within some service branches needs to be achieved. The lack of awareness might be caused by inadequate education or dissemination of the policy, or the confusion caused by apparent conflict with the broader zero tolerance approach.

Of course, the insights from this study need to be considered in light of the study's limitations, particularly the limitations that we noted in the systematic review, including the lack of extensive evidence about effective strategies for preventing and identifying PDM, the use of a limited sample of military medical providers and MTFs, and missing information to complete the mathematical model. It is important to note that we base our recommendations entirely on our review of publicly available materials and hence might miss relevant restricted directives or guidelines that the military uses that speak to some of the points raised here. Before of any of the study's key policy implications can be acted on, it might be wise to conduct a more comprehensive survey of military health providers to obtain more-generalizable data on perspectives, practices, challenges, and recommendations, which can explore whether important differences exist across regions, military facilities, and provider types.

Key-Word Literature Searches

This appendix lists the searches we conducted for PDM prevention and treatment, respectively, in each database.

Prescription Drug Misuse: Prevention

Searches run September 4–5, 2012

PubMed

((abuse[Title/Abstract] OR misuse[Title/Abstract] OR "nonmedical use"[Title/Abstract] OR "non-medical use"[Title/Abstract] OR "non medical use"[Title/Abstract] OR addiction[Title/Abstract] OR dependence[Title/Abstract] OR use[Title/Abstract]
AND
"motivational interviewing"[Title/Abstract] OR prevention[Title/Abstract] OR "brief intervention"[Title/Abstract] OR sbirt[Title/Abstract] OR intervention[Title/Abstract] OR screening[Title/Abstract] OR testing[Title/Abstract] OR policy[Title/Abstract] OR guideline[Title/Abstract] OR "best practice"[Title/Abstract] OR identification[Title/Abstract]
AND
"prescription drug"[Title] OR medication[Title] OR pharmaceutical*[Title] OR stimulant[Title] OR codeine[Title] OR morphine[Title] OR oxycodone[Title] OR oxymorphone[Title] OR hydrocodone[Title] OR hydromorphone[Title] OR benzodiazepine[Title] OR amphetamine*[Title] OR

propoxyphene[Title] OR sedative*[Title] OR hypnotic*[Title]
OR anxiolytic*[Title] OR "opioid analgesic"[Title] OR "opioid
analgesics"[Title] OR z-drug*[Title/Abstract] OR zdrug[Title]
OR "z drug"[Title] OR "z drugs"[Title] OR methadone[Title] OR
buprenorphine[Title] OR medical[Title] OR prescription*[Title]
AND
Substance-related disorders/epidemiology[MeSH] OR
substance-related disorders/prevention & control[MeSH]
AND
Publication date from 2000/01/01; English, Humans))
OR
((abuse[Title/Abstract] OR misuse[Title/Abstract] OR "nonmedical
use"[Title/Abstract] OR "non-medical use"[Title/Abstract] OR
"non medical use"[Title/Abstract] OR addiction[Title/Abstract] OR
dependence[Title/Abstract] OR use[Title/Abstract]
AND
"motivational interviewing"[Title/Abstract] OR prevention[Title/
Abstract] OR "brief intervention"[Title/Abstract] OR sbirt[Title/
Abstract] OR intervention[Title/Abstract] OR screening[Title/
Abstract] OR testing[Title/Abstract] OR policy[Title/Abstract] OR
guideline[Title/Abstract] OR "best practice"[Title/Abstract] OR
identification[Title/Abstract]
AND
"prescription drug"[Title] OR medication[Title] OR
pharmaceutical*[Title] OR stimulant[Title] OR codeine[Title] OR
morphine[Title] OR oxycodone[Title] OR oxymorphone[Title]
OR hydrocodone[Title] OR hydromorphone[Title] OR
benzodiazepine[Title] OR amphetamine*[Title] OR
propoxyphene[Title] OR sedative*[Title] OR hypnotic*[Title]
OR anxiolytic*[Title] OR "opioid analgesic"[Title] OR "opioid
analgesics"[Title] OR z-drug*[Title/Abstract] OR zdrug[Title]
OR "z drug"[Title] OR "z drugs"[Title] OR methadone[Title] OR
buprenorphine[Title] OR medical[Title] OR prescription*[Title]
AND
Publication date from 2000/01/01; English
AND

premedline OR "in process"[sb] OR publisher[sb]))
AND NOT
Monkey[text word] OR Monkeys[text word] OR dog[text word] OR
dogs[Text word] OR rat[text word] OR rats[text word] OR pig[text
word] OR pigs[text word] OR goat[text word] OR goats[text word]
OR "smoking cessation" OR comments[pt] OR editorial[pt] OR case
reports[pt])

Cumulative Index to Nursing and Allied Health Literature
Limiters: Date of Publication from: 20000101-; Language: English;
TI abuse OR TI misuse OR TI "nonmedical use" OR TI
"non-medical use" OR TI "non medical use" OR TI addiction OR
TI dependence OR TI use OR AB abuse OR AB misuse OR AB
"nonmedical use" OR AB "non-medical use" OR AB "non medical
use" OR AB addiction OR AB dependence OR AB use
AND
AB "motivational interviewing" OR AB prevention OR AB "brief
intervention" OR AB sbirt OR AB intervention OR AB screening
OR AB testing OR AB policy OR AB guideline OR AB "best
practice" OR AB identification OR TI "motivational interviewing"
OR TI prevention OR TI "brief intervention" OR TI sbirt OR TI
intervention OR TI screening OR TI testing OR TI policy OR TI
guideline OR TI "best practice" OR TI identification
AND
TI "prescription drug" OR TI medication* OR TI pharmaceutical*
OR TI stimulant* OR TI codeine OR TI morphine OR TI
oxycodone OR TI oxymorphone OR TI hydrocodone OR TI
hydromorphone OR TI benzodiazepine OR TI amphetamine OR TI
propoxyphene OR TI sedative* OR TI hypnotic* OR TI anxiolytic
OR TI "opioid analgesic" OR TI z-drug OR TI zdrug OR TI "z
drug" OR TI methadone OR TI buprenorphine OR TI prescription*
OR TI medical
AND
(MH "Substance Use Disorders+")

EconLit

Limiters: Date of Publication from: 20000101-; Language: English; Publication Type: Journal Article

TI abuse OR TI misuse OR TI "nonmedical use" OR TI "non-medical use" OR TI "non medical use" OR TI addiction OR TI dependence OR TI use OR AB abuse OR AB misuse OR AB "nonmedical use" OR AB "non-medical use" OR AB "non medical use" OR AB addiction OR AB dependence OR AB use
AND
AB "motivational interviewing" OR AB prevention OR AB "brief intervention" OR AB sbirt OR AB intervention OR AB screening OR AB testing OR AB policy OR AB guideline OR AB "best practice" OR AB identification OR TI "motivational interviewing" OR TI prevention OR TI "brief intervention" OR TI sbirt OR TI intervention OR TI screening OR TI testing OR TI policy OR TI guideline OR TI "best practice" OR TI identification
AND
TI "prescription drug" OR TI medication* OR TI pharmaceutical* OR TI stimulant* OR TI codeine OR TI morphine OR TI oxycodone OR TI oxymorphone OR TI hydrocodone OR TI hydromorphone OR TI benzodiazepine OR TI amphetamine OR TI propoxyphene OR TI sedative* OR TI hypnotic* OR TI anxiolytic OR TI "opioid analgesic" OR TI z-drug OR TI zdrug OR TI "z drug" OR TI methadone OR TI buprenorphine OR TI prescription* OR TI medical

PsycInfo

Limiters: Publication Year from: 2000-; Publication Type: All Journals; English;

TI abuse OR TI misuse OR TI "nonmedical use" OR TI "non-medical use" OR TI "non medical use" OR TI addiction OR TI dependence OR TI use OR AB abuse OR AB misuse OR AB "nonmedical use" OR AB "non-medical use" OR AB "non medical use" OR AB addiction OR AB dependence OR AB use
AND

AB "motivational interviewing" OR AB prevention OR AB "brief intervention" OR AB sbirt OR AB intervention OR AB screening OR AB testing OR AB policy OR AB guideline OR AB "best practice" OR AB identification OR TI "motivational interviewing" OR TI prevention OR TI "brief intervention" OR TI sbirt OR TI intervention OR TI screening OR TI testing OR TI policy OR TI guideline OR TI "best practice" OR TI identification
AND
TI "prescription drug" OR TI medication* OR TI pharmaceutical* OR TI stimulant* OR TI codeine OR TI morphine OR TI oxycodone OR TI oxymorphone OR TI hydrocodone OR TI hydromorphone OR TI benzodiazepine OR TI amphetamine OR TI propoxyphene OR TI sedative* OR TI hypnotic* OR TI anxiolytic OR TI "opioid analgesic" OR TI z-drug OR TI zdrug OR TI "z drug" OR TI methadone OR TI buprenorphine OR TI prescription* OR TI medical
AND
DE Drug Abuse OR DE Drug Abuse prevention

Academic Search Complete
Limiters: Published Date from: 20000101-;Language: English
TI abuse OR TI misuse OR TI "nonmedical use" OR TI "non-medical use" OR TI "non medical use" OR TI addiction OR TI dependence OR TI use OR AB abuse OR AB misuse OR AB "nonmedical use" OR AB "non-medical use" OR AB "non medical use" OR AB addiction OR AB dependence OR AB use
AND
AB "motivational interviewing" OR AB prevention OR AB "brief intervention" OR AB sbirt OR AB intervention OR AB screening OR AB testing OR AB policy OR AB guideline OR AB "best practice" OR AB identification OR TI "motivational interviewing" OR TI prevention OR TI "brief intervention" OR TI sbirt OR TI intervention OR TI screening OR TI testing OR TI policy OR TI guideline OR TI "best practice" OR TI identification
AND

TI "prescription drug" OR TI medication* OR TI pharmaceutical*
OR TI stimulant* OR TI codeine OR TI morphine OR TI
oxycodone OR TI oxymorphone OR TI hydrocodone OR TI
hydromorphone OR TI benzodiazepine OR TI amphetamine OR TI
propoxyphene OR TI sedative* OR TI hypnotic* OR TI anxiolytic
OR TI "opioid analgesic" OR TI z-drug OR TI zdrug OR TI "z
drug" OR TI methadone OR TI buprenorphine OR TI prescription*
OR TI medical
AND
((DE "MEDICATION abuse" OR DE "BENZODIAZEPINE
abuse" OR DE "METHAQUALONE abuse" OR DE
"OXYCODONE abuse") OR (DE "SELF medication" OR DE
"MEDICATION abuse" OR DE "MEDICATION errors" OR DE
"PATIENT-controlled analgesia")) OR (DE "OPIOID abuse")

Embase
abuse:ab,ti OR misuse:ab,ti OR 'nonmedical use':ab,ti OR
'non-medical use':ab,ti OR 'non medical use':ab,ti OR addiction:ab,ti
OR dependence:ab,ti AND [humans]/lim AND [english]/lim AND
[embase]/lim AND [2000-2013]/py (removed "use" from this string)
AND
'motivational interviewing':ab,ti OR prevention:ab,ti OR 'brief
intervention':ab,ti OR sbirt:ab,ti OR intervention:ab,ti OR
screening:ab,ti OR testing:ab,ti OR policy:ab,ti OR guideline:ab,ti
OR 'best practice':ab,ti OR identification:ab,ti AND [humans]/lim
AND [english]/lim AND [embase]/lim AND [2000-2013]/py
AND
'prescription drug':ti OR medication*:ti OR pharmaceutical*:ti
OR stimulant*:ti OR codeine:ti OR morphine:ti OR oxycodone:ti
OR oxymorphone:ti OR hydrocodone:ti OR hydromorphone:ti
OR benzodiazepine:ti OR amphetamine*:ti OR propoxyphene:ti
OR sedative*:ti OR hypnotic*:ti OR anxiolytic:ti OR 'opioid
analgesic':ti OR 'opioid analgesics':ti OR zdrug:ti OR 'z drug':ti OR
methadone:ti OR buprenorphine:ti OR medical:ti OR prescription*:ti
AND [humans]/lim AND [english]/lim AND [embase]/lim AND
[2000-2013]/py

Scopus

((((ABS("motivational interviewing") OR ABS(prevention) OR
ABS("brief intervention") OR ABS(sbirt) OR ABS(intervention)
OR ABS(screening) OR ABS(testing) OR ABS(policy) OR
ABS(guideline*) OR ABS("best practice") OR ABS(identification))
AND PUBYEAR > 1999) OR ((TITLE("motivational interviewing")
OR TITLE(prevention) OR TITLE("brief intervention") OR
TITLE(sbirt) OR TITLE(intervention) OR TITLE(screening) OR
TITLE(testing) OR TITLE(policy) OR TITLE(guideline*) OR
TITLE("best practice") OR TITLE(identification)) AND PUBYEAR
> 1999))
AND
((((TITLE(abuse) OR TITLE(misuse) OR TITLE("nonmedical use")
OR TITLE("non-medical use") OR TITLE("non medical use")
OR TITLE(addiction) OR TITLE(dependence)) AND PUBYEAR
> 1999) OR ((ABS(abuse) OR ABS(misuse) OR ABS("nonmedical
use") OR ABS("non-medical use") OR ABS("non medical use") OR
ABS(addiction) OR ABS(dependence)) AND PUBYEAR > 1999))
(removed "use" from this string)
AND
(((TITLE("prescription drug" OR "prescription drugs" OR
medication* OR pharmaceutical* OR stimulant* OR codeine OR
morphine OR oxycodone OR oxymorphone OR hydrocodone
OR thydromorphone OR benzodiazepine* OR amphetamine*
OR propoxyphene OR sedative* OR hypnotic*) AND PUBYEAR
> 1999) OR (TITLE(anxiolytic OR "opioid analgesic" OR
"opioid analgesics" OR zdrug OR "z drug" OR methadone OR
buprenorphine OR medical OR prescription*) AND PUBYEAR >
1999))
Limit to English
AND NOT
(TITLE-ABS-KEY("Smoking cessation"))) AND NOT
(TITLE-ABS-KEY(asthma))) AND NOT (ABS(hiv))) AND NOT
(ABS(monkey OR monkeys OR rat OR rats OR mouse OR mice OR
pig OR pigs)) AND (LIMIT-TO(LANGUAGE, "English"))

Cochrane Database of Systematic Review

From 2000 to 2012

(abuse OR misuse OR "nonmedical use" OR "non-medical use" OR "non medical use" OR addiction OR dependence OR use):ab or (abuse OR misuse OR "nonmedical use" OR "non-medical use" OR "non medical use" OR addiction OR dependence OR use):ti, from 2000 to 2012 in Cochrane Reviews and Other Reviews

AND

"prescription drug" OR "prescription drugs" OR medication* OR pharmaceutical* OR stimulant* OR codeine OR morphine OR oxycodone OR oxymorphone OR hydrocodone OR thydromorphone OR benzodiazepine* OR amphetamine* OR propoxyphene OR sedative* OR hypnotic* OR anxiolytic OR "opioid analgesic" OR "opioid analgesics" OR zdrug OR "z drug" OR methadone OR buprenorphine OR medical OR prescription* :ti, from 2000 to 2012 in Cochrane Reviews and Other Reviews

AND

"motivational interviewing" OR prevention OR "brief intervention" OR sbirt OR intervention OR screening OR testing OR policy OR guideline OR "best practice" OR identification:ab or "motivational interviewing" OR prevention OR "brief intervention" OR sbirt OR intervention OR screening OR testing OR policy OR guideline OR "best practice" OR identification:ti, from 2000 to 2012 in Cochrane Reviews and Other Reviews

Sociological Abstracts

Limits: 2000-; English; Scholarly journals

(ti(abuse OR misuse OR "nonmedical use" OR "non-medical use" OR "non medical use" OR addiction OR dependence OR use) OR ab(abuse OR misuse OR "nonmedical use" OR "non-medical use" OR "non medical use" OR addiction OR dependence OR use))

AND

ti("prescription drug" OR "prescription drugs*" OR medication* OR pharmaceutical* OR stimulant* OR codeine OR morphine OR oxycodone OR oxymorphone OR hydrocodone OR thydromorphone OR benzodiazepine OR amphetamine* OR propoxyphene OR

sedative* OR hypnotic* OR anxiolytic OR "opioid analgesic" OR
"opioid analgesics" OR zdrug OR "z drug" OR methadone OR
buprenorphine OR medical OR prescription*)
AND
(ab("motivational interviewing" OR prevention OR "brief
intervention" OR sbirt OR intervention OR screening OR testing
OR policy OR guideline OR "best practice" OR identification) OR
ti("motivational interviewing" OR prevention OR "brief intervention"
OR sbirt OR intervention OR screening OR testing OR policy OR
guideline OR "best practice" OR identification))

Web of Science

Title=(("prescription drug" OR "prescription drugs*" OR medication*
OR pharmaceutical* OR stimulant* OR codeine OR morphine OR
oxycodone OR oxymorphone OR hydrocodone OR thydromorphone
OR benzodiazepine OR amphetamine* OR propoxyphene OR
sedative* OR hypnotic* OR anxiolytic OR "opioid analgesic" OR
"opioid analgesics" OR zdrug OR "z drug" OR methadone OR
buprenorphine OR medical OR prescription*))
AND
Topic=(abuse OR misuse OR "nonmedical use" OR "non-medical
use" OR "non medical use" OR addiction OR dependence)
AND
Topic=("motivational interviewing" OR prevention OR "brief
intervention" OR sbirt OR intervention OR screening OR testing OR
policy OR guideline OR "best practice" OR identification)
Timespan=2000-01-01
AND TOPIC = Substance Abuse

Prescription Drug Misuse: Treatment

Searches run September 7, 2012

PubMed

"prescription drug"[Title] OR medication[Title] OR pharmaceutical*[Title] OR stimulant[Title] OR codeine[Title] OR morphine[Title] OR oxycodone[Title] OR oxymorphone[Title] OR hydrocodone[Title] OR hydromorphone[Title] OR benzodiazepine[Title] OR amphetamine*[Title] OR propoxyphene[Title] OR sedative*[Title] OR hypnotic*[Title] OR anxiolytic*[Title] OR "opioid analgesic"[Title] OR "opioid analgesics"[Title] OR z-drug*[Title/Abstract] OR zdrug[Title] OR "z drug"[Title] OR "z drugs"[Title] OR methadone[Title] OR buprenorphine[Title] OR medical[Title] OR prescription*[Title]
AND
abuse[Title/Abstract] OR misuse[Title/Abstract] OR "nonmedical use"[Title/Abstract] OR "non-medical use"[Title/Abstract] OR "non medical use"[Title/Abstract] OR addiction[Title/Abstract] OR dependence[Title/Abstract] OR use[Title/Abstract]
AND
treatment OR management OR policy OR guideline OR guidelines OR "best practice" OR "best practices"
AND
Publication date from 2000/01/01; English, Humans))
OR
"prescription drug"[Title] OR medication[Title] OR pharmaceutical*[Title] OR stimulant[Title] OR codeine[Title] OR morphine[Title] OR oxycodone[Title] OR oxymorphone[Title] OR hydrocodone[Title] OR hydromorphone[Title] OR benzodiazepine[Title] OR amphetamine*[Title] OR propoxyphene[Title] OR sedative*[Title] OR hypnotic*[Title] OR anxiolytic*[Title] OR "opioid analgesic"[Title] OR "opioid analgesics"[Title] OR z-drug*[Title/Abstract] OR zdrug[Title] OR "z drug"[Title] OR "z drugs"[Title] OR methadone[Title] OR buprenorphine[Title] OR medical[Title] OR prescription*[Title]
AND
abuse[Title/Abstract] OR misuse[Title/Abstract] OR "nonmedical use"[Title/Abstract] OR "non-medical use"[Title/Abstract] OR

"non medical use"[Title/Abstract] OR addiction[Title/Abstract] OR dependence[Title/Abstract] OR use[Title/Abstract]
AND
treatment OR management OR policy OR guideline OR guidelines OR "best practice" OR "best practices"
AND
Publication date from 2000/01/01; English, Humans)
AND
premedline OR "in process"[sb] OR publisher[sb]))
Monkey[text word] OR Monkeys[text word] OR dog[text word] OR dogs[Text word] OR rat[text word] OR rats[text word] OR pig[text word] OR pigs[text word] OR goat[text word] OR goats[text word] OR "smoking cessation" OR comments[pt] OR editorial[pt] OR case reports[pt])

Cumulative Index to Nursing and Allied Health Literature
Limiters: Date of Publication from: 20000101-; Language: English; Exclude Medline; Academic Journals
TI "prescription drug" OR TI medication* OR TI pharmaceutical* OR TI stimulant* OR TI codeine OR TI morphine OR TI oxycodone OR TI oxymorphone OR TI hydrocodone OR TI hydromorphone OR TI benzodiazepine OR TI amphetamine OR TI propoxyphene OR TI sedative* OR TI hypnotic* OR TI anxiolytic OR TI "opioid analgesic" OR TI z-drug OR TI zdrug OR TI "z drug" OR TI methadone OR TI buprenorphine OR TI prescription* OR TI medical
AND
TI abuse OR TI misuse OR TI "nonmedical use" OR TI "non-medical use" OR TI "non medical use" OR TI addiction OR TI dependence OR TI use OR AB abuse OR AB misuse OR AB "nonmedical use" OR AB "non-medical use" OR AB "non medical use" OR AB addiction OR AB dependence OR AB use
AND
treatment OR treat OR management OR policy OR guideline OR guidelines OR "best practice" OR "best practices" OR SBIRT
NOT

"Smoking cessation"

EconLit

Limiters: Date of Publication from: 20000101-; Language: English; Publication Type: Journal Article
TI "prescription drug" OR TI medication* OR TI pharmaceutical* OR TI stimulant* OR TI codeine OR TI morphine OR TI oxycodone OR TI oxymorphone OR TI hydrocodone OR TI hydromorphone OR TI benzodiazepine OR TI amphetamine OR TI propoxyphene OR TI sedative* OR TI hypnotic* OR TI anxiolytic OR TI "opioid analgesic" OR TI z-drug OR TI zdrug OR TI "z drug" OR TI methadone OR TI buprenorphine OR TI prescription* OR TI medical
AND
TI abuse OR TI misuse OR TI "nonmedical use" OR TI "non-medical use" OR TI "non medical use" OR TI addiction OR TI dependence OR TI use OR AB abuse OR AB misuse OR AB "nonmedical use" OR AB "non-medical use" OR AB "non medical use" OR AB addiction OR AB dependence OR AB use
AND
treatment OR treat OR management OR manage OR policy OR guideline OR guidelines OR "best practice" OR "best practices" OR SBIRT

PsycInfo

Limiters: Publication Year from: 2000-; Publication Type: All Journals; English;
TI "prescription drug" OR TI medication* OR TI pharmaceutical* OR TI stimulant* OR TI codeine OR TI morphine OR TI oxycodone OR TI oxymorphone OR TI hydrocodone OR TI hydromorphone OR TI benzodiazepine OR TI amphetamine OR TI propoxyphene OR TI sedative* OR TI hypnotic* OR TI anxiolytic OR TI "opioid analgesic" OR TI z-drug OR TI zdrug OR TI "z drug" OR TI methadone OR TI buprenorphine OR TI prescription* OR TI medical
AND

TI abuse OR TI misuse OR TI "nonmedical use" OR TI
"non-medical use" OR TI "non medical use" OR TI addiction OR
TI dependence OR AB abuse OR AB misuse OR AB "nonmedical
use" OR AB "non-medical use" OR AB "non medical use" OR AB
addiction OR AB dependence OR
AND
treatment OR treat OR management OR manage OR policy OR
guideline OR guidelines OR "best practice" OR "best practices" OR
SBIRT
NOT
MM "smoking cessation"
NOT
AB china OR chinese OR nigeria OR sweden OR Norway OR france
OR french OR canada OR wales OR england OR portulgal OR
denmark OR cuba OR poland OR hungary OR iran OR iraq OR
egypt OR syria OR belgium OR austrailia OR "new zealand" OR
germany OR austria OR solvakia OR japan OR japanese OR india
OR turkey OR AB Israel OR greece OR thailand OR ireland OR
scotland OR "west africa" OR "south africa" OR malaysia OR AB
israel OR AB finland OR bangkock OR bangladesh OR taiwan
NOT
rats OR mice OR mouse

Sociological Abstracts
Limits: 2000-; English; Scholarly journals
(ti(abuse OR misuse OR "nonmedical use" OR "non-medical use"
OR "non medical use" OR addiction OR dependence OR use) OR
ab(abuse OR misuse OR "nonmedical use" OR "non-medical use"
OR "non medical use" OR addiction OR dependence OR use))
AND
ti("prescription drug" OR "prescription drugs*" OR medication*
OR pharmaceutical* OR stimulant* OR codeine OR morphine OR
oxycodone OR oxymorphone OR hydrocodone OR thydromorphone
OR benzodiazepine OR amphetamine* OR propoxyphene OR
sedative* OR hypnotic* OR anxiolytic OR "opioid analgesic" OR

"opioid analgesics" OR zdrug OR "z drug" OR methadone OR
buprenorphine OR medical OR prescription*)
AND
treatment OR treat OR management OR manage OR policy OR
guideline OR guidelines OR "best practice" OR "best practices" OR
SBIRT

Embase

abuse:ab,ti OR misuse:ab,ti OR 'nonmedical use':ab,ti OR
'non-medical use':ab,ti OR 'non medical use':ab,ti OR addiction:ab,ti
OR dependence:ab,ti AND [humans]/lim AND [english]/lim AND
[embase]/lim AND [2000-2013]/py (removed "use" from this string)
AND
treatment OR treat OR management OR manage OR policy OR
guideline OR guidelines OR 'best practice' OR 'best practices' OR
sbirt
AND
'prescription drug':ti OR medication*:ti OR pharmaceutical*:ti
OR stimulant*:ti OR codeine:ti OR morphine:ti OR oxycodone:ti
OR oxymorphone:ti OR hydrocodone:ti OR hydromorphone:ti
OR benzodiazepine:ti OR amphetamine*:ti OR propoxyphene:ti
OR sedative*:ti OR hypnotic*:ti OR anxiolytic:ti OR 'opioid
analgesic':ti OR 'opioid analgesics':ti OR zdrug:ti OR 'z drug':ti OR
methadone:ti OR buprenorphine:ti OR medical:ti OR prescription*:ti
AND [humans]/lim AND [english]/lim AND [embase]/lim AND
[2000-2013]/py
NOT
monkey OR monkeys OR mouse OR mice OR rat OR rats OR
taiwan OR german OR germany OR france OR italy OR nigeria
OR scotland OR ireland OR norway OR belgium OR wales OR
austrialia OR austria OR bangkok OR thailand OR slovakia OR
sweden OR malaysia OR iran OR iraq OR japan OR china OR
chinese OR 'smoking cessation'

Academic Search Complete

Limiters: Published Date from: 20000101-; Publication Type: Periodical, Educational Report, Health Report; Language: English
TI abuse OR TI misuse OR TI "nonmedical use" OR TI "non-medical use" OR TI "non medical use" OR TI addiction OR TI dependence OR TI use OR AB abuse OR AB misuse OR AB "nonmedical use" OR AB "non-medical use" OR AB "non medical use" OR AB addiction OR AB dependence OR AB use
AND
treatment OR treat OR management OR manage OR policy OR guideline OR guidelines OR 'best practice' OR 'best practices' OR sbirt
AND
TI "prescription drug" OR TI medication* OR TI pharmaceutical* OR TI stimulant* OR TI codeine OR TI morphine OR TI oxycodone OR TI oxymorphone OR TI hydrocodone OR TI hydromorphone OR TI benzodiazepine OR TI amphetamine OR TI propoxyphene OR TI sedative* OR TI hypnotic* OR TI anxiolytic OR TI "opioid analgesic" OR TI z-drug OR TI zdrug OR TI "z drug" OR TI methadone OR TI buprenorphine OR TI prescription* OR TI medical
AND
((DE "MEDICATION abuse" OR DE "BENZODIAZEPINE abuse" OR DE "METHAQUALONE abuse" OR DE "OXYCODONE abuse") OR (DE "SELF medication" OR DE "MEDICATION abuse" OR DE "MEDICATION errors" OR DE "PATIENT-controlled analgesia")) OR (DE "OPIOID abuse")
NOT
monkey OR monkeys OR mouse OR mice OR rat OR rats OR taiwan OR german OR germany OR france OR italy OR nigeria OR scotland OR ireland OR norway OR belgium OR wales OR austrialia OR austria OR bangkok OR thailand OR slovakia OR sweden OR malaysia OR iran OR iraq OR japan OR china OR chinese OR 'smoking cessation'

Web of Science

Title=(("prescription drug" OR "prescription drugs*" OR medication* OR pharmaceutical* OR stimulant* OR codeine OR morphine OR oxycodone OR oxymorphone OR hydrocodone OR thydromorphone OR benzodiazepine OR amphetamine* OR propoxyphene OR sedative* OR hypnotic* OR anxiolytic OR "opioid analgesic" OR "opioid analgesics" OR zdrug OR "z drug" OR methadone OR buprenorphine OR medical OR prescription*))
AND
Topic=(abuse OR misuse OR "nonmedical use" OR "non-medical use" OR "non medical use" OR addiction OR dependence)
AND
Topic=(treatment OR treat OR management OR manage OR policy OR guideline OR guidelines OR 'best practice' OR 'best practices' OR sbirt)
Timespan=2000-01-01; article
AND TOPIC = Substance Abuse
NOT
Title=(monkey OR monkeys OR mouse OR mice OR rat OR rats OR taiwan OR german OR germany OR france OR italy OR nigeria OR scotland OR ireland OR norway OR belgium OR wales OR austrialia OR austria OR bangkok OR thailand OR slovakia OR sweden OR malaysia OR iran OR iraq OR japan OR china OR chinese OR Canada OR 'smoking cessation')

Cochrane

From 2000 to 2012
(abuse OR misuse OR "nonmedical use" OR "non-medical use" OR "non medical use" OR addiction OR dependence OR use):ab or
(abuse OR misuse OR "nonmedical use" OR "non-medical use" OR "non medical use" OR addiction OR dependence OR use):ti, from 2000 to 2012 in Cochrane Reviews and Other Reviews
AND
"prescription drug" OR "prescription drugs" OR medication* OR pharmaceutical* OR stimulant* OR codeine OR morphine OR oxycodone OR oxymorphone OR hydrocodone OR thydromorphone

OR benzodiazepine* OR amphetamine* OR propoxyphene OR
sedative* OR hypnotic* OR anxiolytic OR "opioid analgesic" OR
"opioid analgesics" OR zdrug OR "z drug" OR methadone OR
buprenorphine OR medical OR prescription* :ti, from 2000 to 2012
in Cochrane Reviews and Other Reviews
AND treatment OR treat OR management OR manage OR policy
OR guideline OR guidelines OR 'best practice' OR 'best practices'
OR sbirt
from 2000 to 2012 in Cochrane Reviews and Other Reviews

Scopus

((((TITLE("prescription drug" OR "prescription drugs" OR
medication* OR pharmaceutical* OR stimulant* OR codeine OR
morphine OR oxycodone OR oxymorphone OR hydrocodone
OR thydromorphone OR benzodiazepine* OR amphetamine*
OR propoxyphene OR sedative* OR hypnotic*) AND PUBYEAR
> 1999) OR (TITLE(anxiolytic OR "opioid analgesic" OR
"opioid analgesics" OR zdrug OR "z drug" OR methadone OR
buprenorphine OR medical OR prescription*) AND PUBYEAR
> 1999)))) AND (((((TITLE(abuse) OR TITLE(misuse) OR
TITLE("nonmedical use") OR TITLE("non-medical use")
OR TITLE("non medical use") OR TITLE(addiction) OR
TITLE(dependence)) AND PUBYEAR > 1999) OR ((ABS(abuse)
OR ABS(misuse) OR ABS("nonmedical use") OR ABS("non-medical
use") OR ABS("non medical use") OR ABS(addiction) OR
ABS(dependence)) AND PUBYEAR > 1999))) AND (ALL(treatment
OR treat OR management OR manage OR policy OR guideline
OR guidelines OR 'best practice' OR 'best practices' OR sbirt)
AND PUBYEAR > 1999) AND (LIMIT-TO(AFFILCOUNTRY,
"United States")) AND (LIMIT-TO(DOCTYPE, "ar") OR
LIMIT-TO(DOCTYPE, "re")) AND (LIMIT-TO(LANGUAGE,
"English"))AND (LIMIT-TO(AFFILCOUNTRY, "United States"))
AND (LIMIT-TO(DOCTYPE, "ar") OR LIMIT-TO(DOCTYPE,
"re")) AND (LIMIT-TO(LANGUAGE, "English"))

Analytic Tool for Understanding Flow of Prescription Drug Misuse

It is valuable for employers to have tools that can assist in identifying the health risks that their employees face. In the case of PDM among ADSMs, the concern is a matter of not just health risk but also the risk in terms of combat readiness. Thus, understanding the extent of the PDM problem, particularly the prescription opiate problem, is extremely important. Various types of forecasting models, including Markov, population cohort, compartmental, and microsimulation models, are being applied with increasing frequency to track a variety of health behaviors and health events over time for specific or general populations (Rutter, Zaslavsky, and Feuer, 2011; Sonnenberg and Beck, 1993; Weinstein, O'Brien, et al., 2003; Weinstein, Toy, et al., 2001). Indeed, RAND scientists have even developed cohort and dynamic microsimulation models of illicit-drug use for the civilian population (Everingham and Rydell, 1994; Paddock et al., 2012; Rydell, Caulkins, and Everingham, 1996; Rydell and Everingham, 1994), although no previous model has dealt with the difficult problem of PDM. PDM is unique because of the medically indicated channels through which people are exposed to drugs and the huge heterogeneity (i.e., variation) in ways in which people become dependent.

To assist the military in understanding the factors that contribute to trends in PDM among ADSMs, we built an analytic tool that is based on a modeling framework of the PDM problem. Our hope is that this analytic tool can assist in identifying the key factors driving the military problem, which, in turn, can help identify promising practices that are adaptable to the military context to prevent, manage, and treat PDM. In addition to providing military officials with a better understanding of the incidence and prevalence of PDM beyond what can be determined from regular drug testing and occasional survey data, the model can be used to forecast how the incidence and prevalence of PDM will change in the future if current practices stay the course. Thus, the analytic tool should be a valuable resource for planning resources necessary to treat current and future prescription drug misusers within the military.

Perhaps even more important to military officials, however, is the value the analytic tool provides in terms of projecting how PDM could change in response to a change in any of the model assumptions or transition rules, including initiation rates of light drug use among medically indicated and non–medically indicated users, escalation rates from light to heavy use, the rate at which people enter treatment, and the relative effectiveness of treatment (i.e., predictive forecasting). Alternatively, the analytic tool could be constructed so as to individually consider different classes of prescription drugs (e.g., narcotics, stimulants) and then enable the command to better understand the risks of overprescribing, and hence increasing access to, different types of prescription drugs. The analytic tool can be used as both a predictive forecasting model and as a policy assessment tool to predict the extent to which new policy options might influence predicted prevalence and incidence rates.

Because we could not obtain the necessary data to fully parameterize and test the model, we cannot implement the analytic tool ourselves. Nonetheless, we believe that the information contained in this appendix will be adequate to enable someone with technical modeling skills and access to the relevant information to execute the analytic tool and use it to its full advantage. The language used in this appendix is technical in nature, so as to precisely communicate relevant information to the person who could be charged with implementing the tool.

General Modeling Approach

Modeling a diverse population often requires the population to be subdivided into groups according to common key characteristics that are relevant to the health behavior under consideration. We felt that such an approach would be quite useful in case of PDM, in which some patients have medically indicated use for prescription opiates and others do not. In this project, we therefore adopted a *compartmental model* (also known as a *stock and flow model*), in which we subdivided different combinations of clinical states and characteristics of use into compartments, each homogeneous with respect to some specified characteristic (e.g., susceptible ADSM who is prescribed an addictive prescription drug, or ADSM who is diagnosed with PDM and admitted to treatment). This model can be used to describe changes in the number of people in different compartments and the relationships between compartments.

In models of noninfectious diseases, such as a model of the prevalence of chronic kidney disease, compartments can be used to categorize people into groups with commonalities, such as age, stage, and time since diagnosis. Such characteristics ultimately translate to *an expected time of survival common to people belonging to the same compartment*. For example, in the case of chronic kidney disease, someone might be (1) newly diagnosed with early-stage disease, (2) at a given disease stage and having survived beyond a given time, or (3) progressed to end-stage renal disease. Using a compartmental model, we could describe people's transition from one disease compartment (possibly representing a disease stage) to another, with the ultimate aim of modeling historical data so as to "count" future chronic kidney-disease prevalence.

Models can be very complex and can be formulated to include many detailed clinical states. A model might include compartments that stratify the progression of the disease based on comorbidities and other disease (e.g., for chronic kidney disease, comorbidities include diabetes and hypertension). A prime application of a nonlinear, complex model would be the modeling of the long-term dynamics of infectious diseases, such as influenza or the human immunodeficiency virus, in which positive feedback effects in future incidences directly depend on the prevalence of the disease. However, a detailed model with many compartments would require the estimation of more transition rates from data.

Compartmental models are usually formulated to track population *densities* rather than *individuals* in each compartment—for example, the share of a population distribution that meets various criteria defining (say, initiation, then moving to regular use, and then finally abuse and dependence) (Anderson and May, 1992). Therefore, flows from one compartment (initiation) to another (regular use) are continuous rather than compartments being discrete units. This is desirable because these models can be integrated deterministically by solving a set of coupled differential equations describing the rate of change of the population density in each compartment. The solutions to these deterministic equations provide the dynamics in each compartment.

Compartmental models can also be formulated stochastically (Ball, Britton, and Lyne, 2004). However, frequently, when models are done stochastically, particularly under Monte Carlo simulation techniques, they tend to track individuals rather than population densities in order to allow for variability across individuals within a given compartment in some background variables, as well as unpredictable shocks that can influence a given person's behavior.

Variability can come from two different sources in a stochastic model: uncertainty in parameter estimates and uncertainty in the dynamics of the transition (or who transitions). Because variability in the dynamics of who transitions is usually not as large as that attributable to the uncertainty in the parameter values describing the transition rates, it is more important to conduct an uncertainty and sensitivity analysis on the parameter values, which can be done with the deterministic version of the model. Hence, often, researchers will start with a deterministic formulation of a model (e.g., Levy et al., 2011), like we do here.

The Compartmental Model Description

We developed a two-stratum ordinary differential equation model, which we adapted from the simple mover–stayer drug-use epidemic model presented in Rossi, 2002. This model combines a susceptible–infected–susceptible model with a susceptible–infected–recovered model and relies on the light- and heavy-user models that Everingham and Rydell, 1994, pioneered to simulate the dynamics of drug-misuse epidemics.

Population State Variables

The present model consists of 11 compartments across two strata of drug use: medically indicated and non–medically indicated uses of prescription drugs. We define the susceptible population (denoted by S) as those at risk of initiating medical or nonmedical drug use (denoted respectively by S_M and S_R); then $S = S_M + S_R$. Further, we define and denote by I the compartment of unsusceptible and nonusers, which consists of people who never consume any of the drugs of interest in this study.

We also consider two compartments for light and heavy drug users to capture the two stages of hidden drug use, as Behrens, Caulkins, Tragler, Haunschmied, et al., 1999, notes, and we denote these compartments respectively by L_M and H_M, where the subscript M indicates the medical-use stratum. Given the lack of data estimating the proportions of light and heavy nonmedical drug users, we do not split the population of non–medically indicated drug users along stages of drug abuse.

We denote by WT_i and A_i the treatment (i.e., withdrawal) and abstinence (i.e., recovery) stages, respectively, with the subscript i taking the value M for the medical stratum, or R for the nonmedical stratum, to which we refer in this appendix using an R because it is symbolic of recreational use, which is the most common form of non-medical use. Finally, we define and denote by N the compartment of medical users who refuse treatment, which consists of people who are eligible for prescription drugs but who opt out of treatment. Table B.1 provides a description of each population-state variable with its symbol,

Table B.1
Baseline Population Data (Assumed to Be 2011)

Symbol	Description	Estimate	Potential Source
I	Nonusers of prescription drugs		HRBS
N	Eligible medical drug users who refuse treatment		HRBS
S_M	Susceptible medical drug users		TRICARE pharmacy data
S_R	Susceptible nonmedical (recreational) drug users		HRBS
L_M	Light medical drug users	408,656	Jeffery, 2012; IOM, 2012
H_M	Heavy medical drug users	44,902	Jeffery, 2012; IOM, 2012
R	Nonmedical (recreational) drug users	228,405	Jeffery, 2012; IOM, 2012
WT_M	Treated (withdrawn) medical drug users (rehabilitation)		TRICARE
WT_R	Treated (withdrawn) nonmedical (recreational) drug users (rehabilitation)		TRICARE
A_M	Recovered (abstinent) medical drug users		TRICARE
A_R	Recovered (abstinent) nonmedical (recreational) drug users		TRICARE
K	Total active-duty personnel	1,417,370	IOM, 2012

as well as one potential source of data, although other sources of data might be readily available to those within the military.

Figure B.1 represents the complete state diagram. The arrows on the diagram indicate the directions of the flows between adjacent compartments, and the associated parameters indicate the rates of flow between them. The differential equations characterizing this dynamic are as follows:[1]

---

[1]   In Equations B.1 to B.11, we are using the notation that $\dot{X}(t) = \dfrac{dX(t)}{dt}$.

$$\dot{I}(t) = \alpha_I + \iota N(t) - (\xi + \mu_I) I(t). \tag{B.1}$$

$$\dot{S}_M(t) = \alpha_{SM} + \chi_M A_M(t) + \xi I(t) \\ - (\rho + \gamma_M + \mu_{SM}) S_M(t). \tag{B.2}$$

$$\dot{S}_R(t) = \alpha_{SR} + \chi_R A_R(t) - (\gamma_R + \mu_{SR}) S_R(t). \tag{B.3}$$

$$\dot{R}(t) = \gamma_R S_R(t) - (\psi_R + \mu_R) R(t). \tag{B.4}$$

$$\dot{N}(t) = \rho S_M(t) - (\theta + \iota + \mu_N) N(t). \tag{B.5}$$

$$\dot{L}_M(t) = \gamma_M S_M(t) + \theta N(t) - (\delta + \sigma_M + \mu_{LM}) L_M(t). \tag{B.6}$$

$$\dot{H}_M(t) = \delta L_M(t) - (\psi_M + \mu_{HM}) H_M(t). \tag{B.7}$$

$$\dot{A}_M(t) = \sigma_M L_M(t) + \pi_M WT_M(t) + \nu A_R(t) \\ - (\chi_M + \omega + \mu_{AM}) A_M(t). \tag{B.8}$$

$$\dot{A}_R(t) = \pi_R WT_R(t) + \omega A_M(t) \\ - (\chi_R + \nu + \mu_{AR}) A_R(t). \tag{B.9}$$

$$\dot{WT}_M(t) = \psi_M H_M(t) - (\pi_M + \mu_{WTM}) WT_M(t). \tag{B.10}$$

$$\dot{WT}_R(t) = \psi_R R(t) - (\pi_R + \mu_{WTR}) WT_R(t). \tag{B.11}$$

Model Parameters

We classify the parameter set under three broad categories:

- *Demographic* parameters are related to the overall population changes, in the absence of PDM epidemic, and include chiefly the "military recruitment" and "death" or "dismissal" rates in the population.
    - α_I, α_{SM}, and α_{SR} represent the natural growth rate of non-user, susceptible medical, and susceptible recreational drug user populations, respectively.
    - These parameters can be interpreted as the recruiting rate of new military personnel, weighted by the probabilities η_I, η_{SM}, and η_{SR} that they fall into these compartments.
    - We define the μ_j parameters as the attrition rate (i.e., death rate or rate of dismissal from military service) in any given compartment j.
- *Biological* or *behavioral* parameters are those that capture biological susceptibilities to addiction or behavioral choices to use to the point of dependence, thereby influencing likelihood of initiation, transitioning to heavy use, and difficulty with recovery.
    - γ_M, for example, is the rate at which someone who is using prescription drugs for medicinal purposes transitions into light nonmedical use. This could be influenced by a biological susceptibility to addiction or simply a behavioral choice. γ_R refers to someone who is susceptible to using drugs choosing to initiate prescription drug use recreationally, without a prescription from a doctor.
    - The parameter ξ denotes the rate at which people who stop taking prescription drugs medically (and hence become nonusers, I) return to the susceptible pool, S_M, in which their susceptibility is defined by their previous medical exposure.

Figure B.1
Flow Diagram for an Epidemic of Prescription Drug Misuse

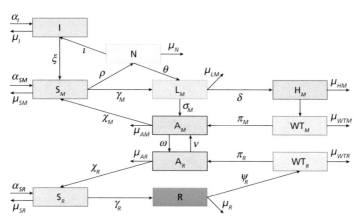

NOTE: The model starts by identifying three types of people: those who will never use a prescription unless they must for medical purposes but even then will not become addicted (I), those who are susceptible to addition or misuse but are first introduced via a legitimate medical need (S_M), and those who are susceptible to addiction or misuse and are first introduced because of a desire to use nonmedically (recreationally). The arrows indicate the directions of the flows between adjacent compartments, and the associated parameters indicate the rates of flow between them. α_I, α_{SM}, and α_{SR} = the natural growth rate of nonuser, susceptible medical, and susceptible recreational drug user populations, respectively. μ_j = the attrition rates in any given compartment j. ξ = the rate at which nonusers of prescription drugs (i.e., those in I) become susceptible to use because of being medically prescribed an addictive substance (S_M). ρ = the rate at which people eligible for medical drug use opt out of treatment. Such individuals might become nonusers of prescription drugs and thus transition to compartment I at the rate ι. γ_M and γ_R = the initiation rates of light drug use among the susceptible medical users and recreational users, respectively. δ = the average rates at which light users escalate to heavy use (H_M). χ_M and χ_R = the rate at which abstinent people in the M and R strata become susceptible to medical and recreational drug use, respectively. σ_M = the average rate at which light users quit drug use to become abstinent. ψ_M and ψ_R = the rates at which heavy and recreational drug users, respectively, initiate treatment. π_M and π_R = the average rates at which people undergoing treatment in the two strata M and R, respectively, become abstinent. ω and v = the switching rates between the two abstinent types.
RAND RR1345-3.1

- The parameters π_M and π_R are the average rates at which people undergoing treatment in the two strata M and R become abstinent.
- We denote by δ the average rates at which light users who are biologically susceptible to addiction escalate to heavy use (H_M).

- The parameter σ_M denotes the average rate at which light users quit drug use to become abstinent.
- We define χ_M and χ_R to denote the rate at which abstinent people in the M and R strata, respectively, become susceptible to medical and recreational drug use. The parameters ω and ν denote the switching rates between the two abstinent types.
- We define ρ to be the rate at which people who would never be susceptible to addiction transition from legitimate medical use of a prescription drug back to the nonuse state.
- *Intervention* parameters are related to the rate at which patients initiate rehabilitation or some form of management of their addiction.
  - We define the parameters ψ_M and ψ_R to represent the rates at which heavy and recreational drug users, respectively, initiate treatment.
  - Because it is feasible that people not susceptible to prescription drug addiction (nonusers, N) might decide to use leftover pain medication given to them for an old injury for a new injury without explicit doctor recommendation, we have a transition value, θ. Because this meets the technical definition of prescription drug misuse but is an accurate reflection of reality that policy interventions could target, we include it.

The model formulated by Equations B.1–B.11 and illustrated in Figure B.1 is a more complicated version of the one shown in Figure 3.1 in Chapter Three. In particular, the model described in this appendix considers some extra processes that Figure 3.1 does not illustrate. Specifically, Figure 3.1 does not show the underlying attrition rates from each compartment that the μ_j parameters represent in Figure B.1. Moreover, Figure 3.1 does not consider the processes that the parameters ξ, ρ, ι, θ, χ_M, χ_R, ω, and ν describe. Therefore, the model described in this appendix can be made to exactly match the model shown in Figure 3.1 by setting these parameter values to 0.

Underlying Model Assumptions

The model relies on several simplifying behavioral and biological assumptions about the prescription drug epidemic. Behaviorally, we assume that people's transition rates from one PDM state to another can be described by population-level averages, and we assume that people do not influence each other's drug-use behaviors. As formulated, our model is linear because it assumes that PDM in the military is a behavior that can lead to termination of someone's contract, and hence there is too great of a risk of getting in trouble if someone tries to use peer pressure to get others to engage in the behavior. However, what that means in the model is that the transitions of a representative person between epidemic states do not depend on any of the epidemic state prevalences. This might be an oversimplifying assumption that can be formally tested once the model is parameterized.

Our model assumes that, unlike heavy medical users, light medical users can transition to the recovered-medical-user stage (i.e., become abstainers) without the aid of treatment. In reality, some heavy medical users could also become abstainers without the aid of treatment; however, this is likely to occur considerably less frequently, which made us neglect this process. Our model further assumes that people in the recovered-medical-user stage can transition to and from recovered non-medical user. Technically, without this process, the model would be split between medical users and nonmedical users with no possibility for service members to transition from one type to the other. We could have assumed that susceptible medical users and susceptible nonmedical users could transition to and from each other's states. However, we assume that people who have never made use of these drugs are of two types only—namely, susceptible medical users and susceptible nonmedical users. People who become susceptible nonmedical users can do so only if they were medical users in the past and had at some point become recovered medical users.

Furthermore, as formulated and described above, our model considers just one population stratum. The model can easily be extended to consider a population stratified over various demographic indicators, such as age group, service branch, rank, or gender. Some of the values of the model parameters describing transition rates would depend on the specific combination of demographic indicators. Quantifying this dependence would require large data sets that include these demographic indicators; the estimation would also require statistical regression analyses. Alternatively, this dependence might be quantified or estimated based on previous studies in the literature. Given the difficulty in identifying and accessing data sets that contain the required information for such an analysis, we opted to proceed with a single-population-stratum model.

Model Integration

Because the model is linear, it can be integrated analytically. An analytical solution is desirable because outputs can be computed more rapidly than in a numerical solution. At the end of this appendix, we provide the analytic solution to our model equations (Equations B.1 to B.11). To verify our solution, we numerically simulated the course of the epidemic using a range of mathematically reasonable (but completely made-up) parameter values and initial conditions and compared simulation results with those obtained by our analytic solution. As expected, results obtained by our analytic solution perfectly matched those obtained by our numerical integration.

Estimation of Parameter Values

To estimate the parameter values of the model, we would need baseline population data for each compartment. In Table B.1, we provide estimates and sources (along with descriptions) of some of the values for each population-state variable that we used as inputs to the model and present our integrating initial conditions. These values represent year 2010 baseline population value estimates. Unfortunately, we were able to identify baseline population values only for the population compartments representing (1) total active-duty personnel, (2) light medical drug users, (3) heavy medical drug users, and (4) recreational drug users. We are missing estimates of population baseline values for the following:

- nonusers of prescription drugs
- eligible medical drug users who refuse treatment
- susceptible recreational drug users
- treated medical drug users (rehabilitation)
- treated recreational drug users (rehabilitation)
- recovered medical drug users (abstinent)
- recovered recreational drug users (abstinent).

Similar compartment-level data over five to ten years would be needed to calibrate the model. These data might be estimable from surveys conducted among active-duty military forces. Golub and Bennett, 2013, could help confirm and further quantify baseline prevalences. The survey, conducted among veteran service members (N = 269) across various military branches between February 2011 and April 2012, identified the pathways to prescription opioid misuse and the relative population sizes given by iatrogenic, opportunistic, and recreational uses that characterize the level of use.

The tables in the rest of this section summarize the parameters needed for the model parameterization. They also include, at times, possible sources or methods that could be used to identify some of the parameters. For some of the missing estimates, the tables indicate potential ways of estimating these values. For example, time-series data on mortality and population dynamics can be used to estimate the prevalence and incidence in some compartments. Specifically, we can estimate the annual prevalence and incidence for a given compartment through a regression fit, and with some functional assumptions. Thus, we model the prevalence X_t at time t as $f(X_t) = \alpha + \beta t + \varepsilon_t$. Here, ε_t represents a noise-induced (i.e., stochastic) error term. Assuming the exponential growth case, the function $f(\cdot)$ is the log function, so that we estimate $\log(X_t) = \alpha + \beta t + \varepsilon_t$. Then the estimated prevalence for year t is given by the relation $\hat{X}_t = \exp(\hat{\alpha} + \hat{\beta}t)$. The incidence X_t can then estimated as $\tilde{X}_t = (\hat{X}_t \Delta X_t - \hat{X}_{t-1}) + \Delta v_t$, where $\Delta v_t = v_t - v_{t-1}$ is a correction term for inflows and outflows due to death and transitions between compartments.

Other approaches that could prove useful in the estimation of parameters include the method that Briggs, Claxton, and Sculpher,

2006, developed for estimating rates from probabilities using the relationship $p = -\exp(-rt)$, where p denotes the transition probability in a given time period, r the rate, and t the time length. For parameters that cannot be estimated with existing data, a focus group with experts on the subject should be conducted to determine the ranges. The appropriateness of any of these methods depends on the data available to the person actually implementing the model.

Estimation of Demographic Parameter Values

Demographic parameters are related to overall population changes in the absence of the PDM epidemic and include the birth and death rates in the population. We could not quantify these parameters with available data. Thus, in Table B.2, we do not provide any ranges of values.

Estimation of the Biological Parameter Values

We categorize as biological the parameters related to the natural course of the epidemic, such as susceptibility (genetic predisposition) (Bray, Pemberton, Lane, et al., 2010). We documented the proportions of the active-duty personnel (excluding recruits, academy cadets, and people who were absent without leave or incarcerated) who misused prescription drugs in 2002 (1.8 percent), 2005 (3.8 percent), and 2008 (11.1 percent). As before, we can estimate the annual misuse through a regression fit and assume the exponential growth case function. The choice of an exponential fit can be justified because, as we note in "Additional Material" at the end of this appendix, the model is linear and thus conforms to the class of exponential population growth models. Thus, as before, the function $f(\cdot)$ is the inverse of the exponential growth (i.e., the log function). We ran an ordinary least squares regression of the log values of these estimates of misuse rates on the year variables:

$$\log[hu_t] = \alpha + \beta t + \varepsilon_t, \tag{B.12}$$

where hu_t denotes the proportion of misuse out of the total number of people in year t and ε_t represents a noise-induced error term. Using the estimated coefficient $\hat{\beta}$ from this regression, we predicted the misuse rates for the years 2011 and 2012. The estimates $\widehat{hu}_t = \exp\left(\hat{\alpha} + \hat{\beta}t\right)$

Table B.2
Demographic Parameters

Symbol	Parameter Description	Potential Source
α	Recruiting rate (growth rate)	Defense Enrollment Eligibility Reporting System, census
η_I	Risk of no drug use	Testing data (proportion clean), HRBS
η_{SM}	Risk of medical drug use	TRICARE data (proportion of active enrollees who are prescribed a drug), HRBS
η_{SR}	Risk of recreational use	Calculated: $1 - \left(\eta_I + \eta_{SM} \right)$
α_I	Rate of growth of the nonusers	Calculated: $\eta_I \times \alpha$
α_{SM}	Rate of growth of the medical users	Calculated: $\eta_{SM} \times \alpha$
α_{SR}	Rate of growth of the recreational users	Calculated: $\eta_{SR} \times \alpha$
μ_X	Rate of death and dismissal from the services from X	Defense Enrollment Eligibility Reporting System

and $\Delta h\tilde{u}_t = \widehat{uh}_{t-1} - \widehat{hu}_t$ represent, respectively, the total prevalence and total incidence of drug misuse during year t as a proportion of the total population. Therefore, we can think of $\hat{h}_t$ as an estimate of the ratio of the number of people HU_t to the total number of people K_t, where

$$HU_t = L_{M,t} + H_{M,t} + R_t \tag{B.13}$$

and

$$K_t = HU_t + I_t + N_t + S_{M,t} + S_{R,t} \\ + A_{M,t} + A_{R,t} + WT_{M,t} + WT_{R,t}. \tag{B.14}$$

Similarly, Δh_t estimates the incidence of misuse for the joint L_M, H_M, and R compartments, so that

$$\Delta h_t K_t = \gamma_M S_{M,t} + \theta N_t + \gamma_R S_{R,t}. \tag{B.15}$$

We can more reliably estimate γ_R as opposed to γ_M and θ from the literature. For example, Behrens, Caulkins, Tragler, Haunschmied, et al., 1999, estimates the average rate at which light users attract non-users to be $s = 0.61$ in a study of cocaine initiation. Because those using medical drugs for recreational purposes will likely be more similar to illegal-drug users than the medical users would be, we can estimate γ_R by s. If we define θ^f such that $\theta = \theta^f \gamma_M$, then γ_M and θ can be estimated by

$$\hat{\gamma}_M = \frac{E[\tilde{u}_t K_t] - \gamma_R E[S_{R,t}]}{E[S_{M,t}] + \theta^f E[N_t]} \frac{\Delta h_t E[\tilde{u}_t K_t] - \gamma_R E[S_{R,t}]}{E[S_{M,t}] + \theta^f E[N_t]},$$

and

$$\hat{\theta} = \theta^f \hat{\gamma}_M. \tag{B.16}$$

Therefore, instead of estimating $\hat{\gamma}_M$ and θ separately, we assume a function (i.e., multiplication by θ^f) that links the two. Therefore, our estimate for $\hat{\gamma}_M$ allows us to estimate θ. Table B.3 summarizes descriptively the biological parameters used in the model, along with their sources. Most parameters are rates and thus have units of inverse years.

Estimation of Behavioral Parameter Values

Behavioral parameters are related to people's choices and decisions, such as the rate of initiation of drug use. In the model, the key behavioral parameters are ρ, which indicates the refusal rate of treatment for eligible patients; γ_R, which is the initiation rate of recreational drug use; and ω, which is the switching rate from medical to recreational drug use. Starting values for these parameters could come from the literature or available data in the military, such as the HRBS. Policy

Table B.3
Biological Parameters for the Model

Symbol	Parameter Description	Value			Potential Source
		Median	Lower	Upper	
ξ	Rate of becoming susceptible for nonusers	—	—	—	Assumption
ι	Rate of becoming nonuser for refusers	—	—	—	Assumption
γ_M	Initiation rate of light drug use	0.36	0.10	1.61	Estimated (National Survey on Drug Use and Health)
π_M	Recovery rate of treated medical user	0.47	0.75	1.00	IOM, 2012
π_R^f	Multiplicative factor for recovery rate	1.00	—	—	Assumption
π_R	Recovery rate of treated recreational users	0.47	0.75	1.00	Calculated: $\pi_R^f \pi_M$
β	Multiplicative factor for initiation rate	—	—	—	Assumption
δ	Initiation rate of heavy drug use	—	—	—	Calculated: $\beta \gamma_M$
σ_M	Rate at which light drug users become abstinent	0.35	—	—	IOM, 2012
ν	Switching rate from recreational to medical drug use	—	—	—	Assumption

interventions could target such parameters in order to affect the course of the epidemic.

Estimation of Intervention Parameter Values

Intervention parameters are related to the rate at which patients initiate rehabilitation or some form of treatment for their addictions. Table B.4 provides some ideas of potential sources for constructing estimates, based on our knowledge of the literature.

Table B.4
Some Potential Sources for Intervention Parameter Values

Symbol	Parameter Description	Potential Source
θ^f	Multiplicative factor for light drug use initiation	Calculate from World Wide Survey on Health Related Behaviors or National Survey on Drug Use and Health
θ	Initiation rate of light drug use among nonusers	Calculated: $\theta^f \gamma_M$
ψ_M	Rate of treatment initiation among medical drug users	Calculate from the Treatment Episode Data Set
ψ_R	Rate of treatment initiation among recreational drug users	Calculate from the Treatment Episode Data Set

Model Calibration, Uncertainty, and Sensitivity Analyses

As described earlier, because we lack available data sets, we could not quantify many of the model parameters and the baseline population representing our initial conditions for the model integration. Consequently, we could not run our model and complete its analyses. In this section, we describe the model calibration process and model sensitivity analysis that we would have carried out if we had estimates for all model parameter values and their uncertainty ranges. Model calibration and sensitivity analysis are necessary steps that are done before using the model as a prediction tool. Without model calibration, it is not possible to assess whether predictions made with the model are reasonable or robust. Nevertheless, an uncalibrated model also has its uses. For example, application of uncalibrated models can be very useful in guiding data-collection activities.

Model calibration consists of changing values of model input parameters in an attempt to match the observed steady state or the observed dynamics of the population state variable relative to some acceptable criteria, known as tolerance. When calibrating the model to the steady state, it is assumed that the prevalences for each population compartment are time-invariant. If this latter assumption is true, then the calibration involves searching for combinations of parameter values that are consistent with the steady state prevalences. Unique combinations of parameter values can be generated efficiently via a Latin hypercube sampling procedure (Hoare, Regan, and Wilson, 2008), which is a statistical method for generating a sample of plausible collections of parameter values from a multidimensional distribution. We can generate hundreds of thousands of unique parameter value combinations by assuming that each model parameter falls within its specified uncertainty range, according to some assumed probability distribution (e.g., a uniform distribution). We then search for the combination of parameter values that best approximate the analytical solution of our model for the steady state, as given by Equations B.1–B.11. Different criteria can be used to determine the "best" combination of parameter values. No universally accepted goodness-of-fit criteria apply in all cases. We choose the criteria that minimize the sum of the squared differences between the observed and the expected population prevalences and check that this variability is small (i.e., within 5- or 10-percent tolerance range).

If it cannot be assumed that the prevalences have reached their steady states, we would need a time series of observed prevalences for each population compartment over the course of several years. Using the same set of unique combinations of parameter values that our Latin hypercube sampling generated and starting from the initial prevalences given by the data, we can integrate our model forward in time to obtain different realizations for the dynamics of the prevalence of each population compartment. We then need to find the realization that best follows the observed time series of the prevalences given by the data. Again, we base our optimization criteria on finding the realization that yields the smallest sum of the squared differences between the observed and the expected population prevalences over time. This procedure allows us to select the combination of parameter values that is best at reproducing the observed dynamics. However, we also keep all other combinations that produce dynamics within a given threshold from the observed data. As stated earlier, the selected threshold can be 5 or 10 percent. Thus, out of the initial hundreds of thousands of realizations, we filter those that are best at reproducing the observed dynamics.

Good modeling practice requires the modeler to evaluate the confidence in the model. Like the value of any epidemiological model of health behavior, the value of the tool we propose here will depend on the reliability of estimates obtained for the various parameters that make up the model. This evaluation requires, first, a quantification of the level of uncertainty in any model results (i.e., uncertainty analysis), and second, an evaluation of the relative weight or value each input has on the output (i.e., sensitivity analysis). Therefore, using the filtered set of model realizations that we found to best reproduce past observed prevalences, we would conduct both uncertainty and sensitivity analyses of our model. This would require running our model forward in time, as a prediction tool. Therefore, assuming no change in policy or in conditions under which we make our predictions, all parameter values would remain unaltered. We would then run our model using each set of parameter values belonging to the filtered set. Our uncertainty analysis would then assess the variability of our model outputs with respect to the variability of the model inputs. Model outputs we consider here include all the prevalences in each population compartment over time. We would further use our model outputs for our sensitivity analysis. Here we would assess how the uncertainty in the output of our model or system can be apportioned to different sources of uncertainty in the model's input parameters. We would do this by ranking the importance by both strength and relevance of the parameter inputs in determining the variation in the outputs.

Conclusions

It is valuable for any employer to have tools that can assist in identifying the health risks that employees face. In the case of PDM in the military, the concern is a matter of not just health risk but also the risk in terms of combat readiness. Readiness matters not just for individual service members but for their entire units or teams. Thus, understanding the extent of the PDM problem, particularly the prescription opiate problem, is extremely important. Opioids are among the most commonly prescribed medications in the military for pain medication, and recent data suggest that just over one-quarter of ADSMs received at least one prescription for opioids in 2010 (Jeffery, May, et al., 2014). Moreover, another study suggests that two-thirds of those who are identified as prescription opioid misusers began their misuse while on deployment (Golub and Bennett, 2013).

In this appendix, we described an analytic tool that, once parameterized, could serve as a valuable tool for military commanders interested in understanding the dynamics of the current PDM problem. In addition to providing military officials with a better understanding of the incidence and prevalence of PDM beyond what can be determined from regular drug testing and occasional survey data, the model can be used to forecast how the incidence and prevalence of PDM will change in the future if current practices stay the course. Thus, the analytic tool could be very useful for planning resources necessary to treat current and future prescription drug misusers within the military. Perhaps even more important to military officials, however, is the value the analytic tool provides in terms of projecting how PDM could change in response to change in any of the model parameters, including initiation rates of light drug use among medically indicated and non–medically indicated users, escalation rates from light to heavy use, the rate at which people enter treatment, and the relative effectiveness of treatment (predictive forecasting). Alternatively, the analytic tool could be parameterized for different types of prescription drugs (e.g., narcotics, stimulants) and then enable the command to better understand the risks of overprescribing (and hence increasing access) of different types of prescription drugs.

Like the value of any epidemiological model of health behavior, the value of the tool we propose here will depend on the reliability of estimates obtained for the various parameters that make up the model. Our scan of the data fields contained in the TRICARE, HRBS, and drug testing data suggest that sufficient information exists to parameterize the model. Standard techniques for checking reliability and validity of the model would be necessary, but, assuming that the model is shown to be both externally validated and reliable, the tool proposed here could provide military command with good guidance on how to target limited prevention and treatment dollars toward the key parameters that seem to drive higher rates of misuse.

Additional Material: An Analytic Solution to a Prescription Drug Model

The ordinary differential equations presented in Equations B.1–B.11 are simple enough to be solved analytically. In fact, we can rewrite these in matrix form as

$$\dot{X}(t) = K + MX(t), \tag{B.17}$$

where $X(t)$ is a vector of the population state variables,

$$\dot{X}(t) = \frac{dX(t)}{dt}$$

is the vector of the rate of change of $X(t)$, K is also a vector giving the exogenous growth rates, and M is a matrix encapsulates the transition rates to and from the different population compartments. $X(t)$ and K are respectively given by

$$X(t) = \begin{bmatrix} I(t) & S_M(t) & S_R(t) & R(t) & N(t) & L_M(t) \\ H_M(t) & A_M(t) & A_R(t) & WT_M(t) & WT_R(t) \end{bmatrix},$$

and

$$K = \begin{bmatrix} \alpha_I & \alpha_{SM} & \alpha_{SR} & 0 & 0 & 0 & 0 & 0 & 0 & 0 & 0 \end{bmatrix}.$$

The matrix M is given by

$$M = \begin{bmatrix} \zeta_1 & 0 & 0 & \iota & 0 & 0 & 0 & 0 & 0 & 0 & 0 \\ 0 & \zeta_2 & 0 & 0 & 0 & 0 & 0 & \chi_M & 0 & 0 & 0 \\ 0 & 0 & \zeta_3 & 0 & 0 & 0 & 0 & 0 & \chi_R & 0 & 0 \\ 0 & 0 & \gamma_R & \zeta_4 & 0 & 0 & 0 & 0 & 0 & 0 & 0 \\ 0 & \rho & 0 & 0 & \zeta_5 & 0 & 0 & 0 & 0 & 0 & 0 \\ 0 & \gamma_M & 0 & 0 & \theta & \zeta_6 & 0 & 0 & 0 & 0 & 0 \\ 0 & 0 & 0 & 0 & 0 & \delta & \zeta_7 & 0 & 0 & 0 & 0 \\ 0 & 0 & 0 & 0 & 0 & \sigma_M & 0 & \zeta_8 & \nu & \pi_M & 0 \\ 0 & 0 & 0 & 0 & 0 & 0 & 0 & \omega & \zeta_9 & 0 & \pi_R \\ 0 & 0 & 0 & 0 & 0 & 0 & \psi_M & 0 & 0 & \zeta_{10} & 0 \\ 0 & 0 & 0 & \psi_R & 0 & 0 & 0 & 0 & 0 & 0 & \zeta_{11} \end{bmatrix},$$

where

$$\zeta_1 = -\left(\xi + \mu_I\right)$$
$$\zeta_2 = -\left(\rho + \gamma_M + \mu_{SM}\right)$$
$$\zeta_3 = -\left(\gamma_R + \mu_{SR}\right)$$
$$\zeta_4 = -\left(\psi_R + \mu_R\right)$$
$$\zeta_5 = -\left(\theta + \iota + \mu_N\right)$$
$$\zeta_6 = -\left(\delta + \sigma_M + \mu_{LM}\right)$$
$$\zeta_7 = -\left(\psi_M + \mu_{HM}\right)$$
$$\zeta_8 = -\left(\chi_M + \omega + \mu_{AM}\right)$$
$$\zeta_9 = -\left(\gamma_R + \nu + \mu_{AR}\right)$$
$$\zeta_{10} = -\left(\pi_M + \mu_{WTM}\right)$$
$$\zeta_{11} = -\left(\pi_R + \mu_{WTR}\right).$$

We proceed by diagonalization of the matrix M. We thus compute the diagonal matrix Λ containing the eigenvalues of M along the diagonal with all nondiagonal terms at 0. We further compute the matrix B containing the respective eigenvectors of M. Thus we can express M as $M = B\Lambda B^{-1}$. It follows that $M^{-1} = B\Lambda^{-1}B^{-1}$ and $e^{Mt} = Be^{\Lambda t}B^{-1}$, so that

$$\frac{d}{dt}\left[e^{-Mt}\right] = -B\Lambda e^{-\Lambda t}B^{-1} = -Me^{-Mt} = -e^{-Mt}M.$$

(B.18)

Then multiplying both sides of the differential equation by e^{-Mt}, we have

$$e^{-Mt}\dot{X}(t) = e^{-Mt}MX(t) + e^{-Mt}K$$
$$\Rightarrow e^{-Mt}\dot{X}(t) - e^{-Mt}MX(t)$$
$$= e^{-Mt}K$$
$$\Leftrightarrow \frac{d}{dt}\left[e^{-Mt}X(t)\right]$$
$$= e^{-Mt}K$$
$$\Leftrightarrow e^{-Mt}X(t) - X(0)$$
$$= \left(\int_0^t Be^{-\Lambda t}B^{-1}\,dt\right)K$$
$$\Leftrightarrow e^{-Mt}X(t) - X(0)$$
$$= M^{-1}K - M^{-1}e^{-Mt}K.$$

It follows that

$$X(t) = e^{Mt}\left[X(0) + M^{-1}K\right] - e^{Mt}M^{-1}e^{-Mt}K$$
$$= e^{Mt}\left[X(0) + M^{-1}K\right] - M^{-1}K.$$

(B.19)

Existence of a Steady State Equilibrium

Using the analytical solution in Relations B.12–B.14, we can determine the conditions under which a steady state equilibrium is achieved in the system. At the steady state, the total inflows into any state must equal the total outflows from that state. Mathematically, this is formalized by the relation

$$\dot{X}(t) = K + MX(t) = 0. \tag{B.20}$$

Relations B.14 and B.15 imply that $X(0) = -M^{-1}K$ or that t approaches $-\infty$. The first solution is trivial because it implies—using Relation B.14—that $X(t)$ is constant in time. The second solution is simply impossible because time must be positive. Hence, the only steady state equilibrium for this system is the trivial solution.

Tools Used in the Qualitative Interview

In this appendix, we provide the content of the email we sent to commanders and the discussion guide we used for our interviews with key informants. We have not altered the content, only formatted it consistently with the rest of the report.

Email to Base and/or Health Commanders

Dear [name of health commander],

The Deputy Assistant Secretary of Defense for Readiness has engaged the RAND Corporation's National Defense Research Institute (NDRI) in a research project to help estimate the potential burden PDM poses to the military. In order to learn about best practices for identifying and treating the problem, RAND will be conducting in-person interviews at up to 12 military health facilities across the country. We plan to interview medical and behavioral health providers, including emergency room doctors, primary care and family physicians, nurses, medical assistants, pharmacists, and case workers; where possible, we also will interview behavioral health providers in substance use disorder treatment programs.

[Name of MTF] is one of the selected facilities. We are writing to request your assistance accessing a POC within your facility who can help us identify individuals to interview and facilitate scheduling and logistics.

Attached for your reference you will find an OASD [Office of the Assistant Secretary of Defense] memorandum outlining the proposed work and requesting your assistance with our research, as well as a document from OASD indicating exemption of this work from second level review.

At your convenience, please feel free to call me on my office number below or to respond directly to this e-mail. I would greatly appreciate any assistance you can provide.

Sincerely,

RAND Team Member

Key Informant Discussion Guide (5/29/14)

Verbal Consent

Good morning/afternoon/evening. My name is _____, and I am visiting from the RAND Corporation, which is a non-profit organization conducting a research project sponsored by the DoD. The project is examining how PDM impacts the military. (*If appropriate:* (Name) recommended I contact you.) Do you have a few minutes for me to share why I'm visiting today?

[*If yes*] Great, thank you. I'm visiting because we are gathering information about how PDM is identified and treated among active military personnel. We're doing expert interviews and you've been recommended because of the services you provide. The interview would be voluntary and would take about 45 minutes to an hour. We could schedule it at a time convenient for you. Would you be willing to be interviewed?

[*If no*] We terminate the interview.

[If yes: *start interview*] Thank you again for taking the time to speak with me. As a reminder, this project is to examine how PDM is identified, prevented, and treated in the military. You are not required to speak with me, and you can skip any questions you'd like. We'll spend about 45 minutes to an hour today and I'll ask you about three main topics. I'll ask about the current practices and training your department provides in terms of identifying people at risk of misuse and engaging them in treatment, general impressions about PDM, and final recommendations. We ask that you answer these questions as you observe things in your official capacity—we are not asking for personal opinions. How does that sound so far?

In our report, we will summarize our findings from all our interviews and will not label any comments with your name or organization's name, but we may describe the type of organization you represent (for example, military hospital in the Midwest). So, the interview will not be completely anonymous. Is that okay? Do you have any questions?

Great, let's get started then. I'm going to be typing some notes while we talk so that I can capture what you [sic].

Background Info

A Date: _____

B DoD participant ID number: _____

C RAND interviewer: _____

D DoD participant rank: _____

E DoD participant occupation: _____

F DoD participant service branch: _____

General Impressions

1. What are your general impressions about PDM in the military? How has it changed over time? Are there any subgroups that experience this issue more or less? Are your impressions based on your own personal experiences, or based on things you have read or heard from others?
2. Which substances are most commonly misused?
3. Which departments interact most with individuals that misuse prescription drugs?
4. For service members experiencing misuse, how do they access the prescription drugs they are misusing (e.g., do they prescription shop between multiple doctors, go to community-based settings, etc.)?

Current Policies and Procedures

1. First, I'd like to ask you whether there are any formal policies or procedures in place specific to PDM that your department/team has been informed of by the DoD's Health Affairs or another centralized agency? If yes, what are they? (Prompt if necessary: How about for prevention, treatment, medication monitoring?; Prompt if necessary, for each policy mentioned: Is this a DoD policy, a policy specific to your service, or a policy for your installation? Do you know when the policy was established?)

2. How does your department/team put these policies/procedures into action or what gets in the way of implementing these policies/procedures?

3. What other efforts have been made to educate your department/team on what to do when you identify a service member and/or his/her family with a PDM problem (e.g., formal training, official protocols to follow, videos)?

4. How are these policies monitored and/or enforced?

5. How are you informed of any updates or changes in these policies and/or procedures?

Practices

1. Now I'd like to shift to focus specifically on prevention *practices* that might be used to identify or detect someone with a potential PDM problem, such as screening. The DoD guidelines require that active duty be referred to specialty substance use disorder (SUD) care whenever a substance use disorder is suspected. In the [*specific setting: primary care/ER*] setting, do you use a standardized screening tool or procedure (e.g. drug testing) on all patients to identify someone at risk of PDM? If yes, what do you use? If not, how would a provider in your setting come to suspect a PDM problem?

   a. Are these practices different for prescription drug misusers than they are for individuals misusing alcohol or other substances? If so, how?

    b. Do the same procedures /practices apply to high risk patients with chronic pain or a behavioral health issue or are other procedures applied to these high risk groups?

    c. Would you say the procedures/practices used for identifying people at risk are more informal and vary from caregiver to caregiver at this setting, or is there a consistent approach?

    d. How is compliance with following these procedures/practices monitored or updated (e.g., are there audits)?

2. Once a patient is screened positive or identified as "at risk" for PDM, what are the next steps?

    a. Are there clear clinical or department guidelines identifying next steps for your [department] setting?

    b. What are the possible options (e.g. connect immediately to behavioral health services? recommend inpatient/outpatient treatment? assign a case worker? provide counseling? notify patient's chain of command?)

    c. Do those guidelines differ depending on whether the patient is military personnel or a dependent (spouse, child)?

    d. Do those guidelines differ depending on the service branch of the military?

    e. What about if they are on active duty?

3. Now suppose that a service member is identified as being in need of treatment for prescription drug abuse by someone in your setting. In the [*specific setting: primary care/ER*] setting, do medical professionals attempt to treat the service member here? If so, how? If not, what do they do?

    a. For DoD active duty, opioid agonist treatment is not usually an option for treatment according to DoD guidelines. Are you aware of any conditions in which active duty patients might be receiving an opioid agonist treatment (like methadone)? What about buprenorphine/naltrexone?

    b. Are these practices just described followed by all clinical personnel here or is there variance? What factors influence the variance that might occur?

    c. Are these practices formalized in a policy or formal protocol for this department?

      d. If they are adopted as formal policies, how are these policies monitored or enforced (e.g. are there audits)? How frequently?

4. Suppose the service member identified as misusing prescription drugs is someone who was initially given the prescription drug because of a legitimate physical ailment, in particular chronic pain. For a service member experiencing chronic pain due to a severe physical injury or impairment, are there criteria/checks in place for prescribing an opioid-based pain reliever so as to reduce the potential for misuse of the prescription drug?

      a. Are there standard protocols or recommendations for identifying which patients are good candidates for this type of treatment and which patients are bad candidates?

      b. What are the rules for denying someone access to an opioid-based pain reliever?

      c. Are there standard protocols or recommendations for identifying how and when a patient should be tapered off the opioid-based pain reliever? If so, what are they?

      d. How are these prescribing and tapering policies monitored or enforced (e.g., are there audits)?

5. Let's talk about medication monitoring now.

      a. What rules or standard practices are there regarding the numbers of pills that can be prescribed over a given time period when prescribing particular drugs that are highly abused (such as oxycodone, hydrocodone, codeine or benzodiazepines)?

      b. What checks on early or excessive refills are you aware of? How often are these checks used and is information about suspicious behavior by certain patients made available to all providers?

      c. Do these rules or standard practices differ for at-risk populations (e.g. those with chronic pain or mental health issues)?

      d. Are there programs for dispensing of unused medications, so as to avoid access to prescription drugs when they are no longer needed?

Experiences

1. What are challenges you experience when working with service members with PDM issues? How do these differ from individuals with alcohol or illegal drug misuse?
2. How do these challenges compare to other branches of the military or the civilian population?
3. How about the screening and treatment practices we discussed earlier, are they similar or different to those used in the civilian sector?
4. If you were to redesign any of the screening and treatment practices we talked about, what would you do differently?

Training

1. How do you learn about the latest ways to specifically address DPM [sic] (not substance use)? What types of trainings, if any, have you and members in your department [insert prompt with appropriate department: testing, medical, or treatment] received to identify and treat DPM [sic]?
2. Have you been exposed to any training videos specific to PDM? If so, which ones?
    a. How helpful and effective was the training?
    b. Is the training applicable to all services branches or just your own?

Other Recommendations

1. What do you think needs to be done to better address the challenges and barriers we spoke of? [Prompt: List specific challenges/barriers mentioned earlier here]
2. How can identification of and treatment for PDM be improved in the military?
3. What have I missed, what other comments would you like to share?

Bibliography

Agency for Healthcare Research and Quality, "National Guideline Clearinghouse," undated. As of August 18, 2014: http://www.guideline.gov

Air Force Surgeon General, *Guidance Memorandum for Air Force Instruction (AFI) 44-172, Mental Health*, Air Force Instruction 44-172 Air Force Guidance Memorandum 1, September 5, 2012.

Anderson, Roy M., and Robert M. May, *Infectious Diseases of Humans: Dynamics and Control*, Oxford: Oxford University Press, 1992.

Arfken, C. L., C. E. Johanson, S. di Menza, and C. R. Schuster, "Expanding Treatment Capacity for Opioid Dependence with Office-Based Treatment with Buprenorphine: National Surveys of Physicians," *Journal of Substance Abuse Treatment*, Vol. 39, No. 2, September 2010, pp. 96–104.

Assistant Chief of Staff for Health Care Operations, Bureau of Medicine and Surgery, Department of the Navy, *Standards for Provision of Substance Related Disorder Treatment Services*, Bureau of Medicine and Surgery Instruction 5353.4A, November 23, 1999.

Assistant Chief of Staff for Health Policy and Services, Headquarters, U.S. Army Medical Command, *Medical Review Officers and Review of Positive Urinalysis Drug Testing Results*, U.S. Army Medical Command Regulation 40-51, 2011.

Assistant Secretary of Defense for Health Affairs, *Rehabilitation and Referral Services for Alcohol and Drug Abusers*, Department of Defense Instruction 1010.6, March 13, 1985. As of February 27, 2016: https://www.doi.gov/sites/doi.gov/files/migrated/ibc/vendors/upload/D12PS50899_new_Att42.pdf

Assistant Secretary of Defense for Special Operations and Low-Intensity Conflict, *Drug and Alcohol Abuse by DoD Personnel*, Department of Defense Directive 1010.4, September 3, 1997.

———, *Military Personnel Drug Abuse Testing Program*, Department of Defense Directive 1010.1, December 9, 1994, incorporating change 1, January 11, 1999a.

————, *Drug and Alcohol Abuse by DoD Personnel*, Department of Defense Directive 1010.4, September 3, 1997, incorporating change 1, January 11, 1999b.

Assistant Secretary of the Navy for Manpower and Reserve Affairs, *Military Substance Abuse Prevention and Control*, Secretary of the Navy Instruction 5300.28E, May 23, 2011. As of February 27, 2016: http://www.public.navy.mil/surfor/documents/5300_28e.pdf

Baehren, David F., Catherine A. Marco, Danna E. Droz, Sameer Sinha, E. Megan Callan, and Peter Akpunonu, "A Statewide Prescription Monitoring Program Affects Emergency Department Prescribing Behaviors," *Annals of Emergency Medicine*, Vol. 56, No. 1, July 2010, pp. 19–23.

Ball, Frank, Tom Britton, and Owen Lyne, "Stochastic Multitype Epidemics in a Community of Households: Estimation and Form of Optimal Vaccination Schemes," *Mathematical Biosciences*, Vol. 191, No. 1, September 2004, pp. 19–40.

Banta-Green, Caleb J., Charles Maynard, Thomas D. Koepsell, Elizabeth A. Wells, and Dennis M. Donovan, "Retention in Methadone Maintenance Drug Treatment for Prescription-Type Opioid Primary Users Compared to Heroin Users," *Addiction*, Vol. 104, No. 5, May 2009, pp. 775–783.

Barlas, Frances M., William Bryan Higgins, Jacqueline C. Pflieger, and Kelly Diecker, *2011 Health Related Behaviors Survey of Active Duty Military Personnel: Executive Summary*, Washington, D.C.: TRICARE Management Activity and U.S. Coast Guard, February 2013. As of February 25, 2016: http://health.mil/Reference-Center/Reports/2013/02/01/ 2011-Health-Related-Behaviors-Active-Duty-Executive-Summary

Barry, Declan T., Kevin S. Irwin, Emlyn S. Jones, William C. Becker, Jeanette M. Tetrault, Lynn E. Sullivan, Helena Hansen, Patrick G. O'Connor, Richard S. Schottenfeld, and David A. Fiellin, "Integrating Buprenorphine Treatment into Office-Based Practice: A Qualitative Study," *Journal of General Internal Medicine*, Vol. 24, No. 2, February 2009, pp. 218–225.

Behrens, Doris A., Jonathan P. Caulkins, Gernot Tragler, and Gustav Feichtinger, "Optimal Control of Drug Epidemics: Prevent and Treat—but Not at the Same Time?" *Management Science*, Vol. 46, No. 3, March 2000, pp. 333–347.

Behrens, Doris A., Jonathan P. Caulkins, Gernot Tragler, Josef Haunschmied, and Gustav Feichtinger, "A Dynamic Model of Drug Initiation: Implications for Treatment and Drug Control," *Mathematical Biosciences*, Vol. 159, No. 1, June 1999, pp. 1–20.

Belgrade, Miles J., Cassandra D. Schamber, and Bruce R. Lindgren, "The DIRE Score: Predicting Outcomes of Opioid Prescribing for Chronic Pain," *Journal of Pain*, Vol. 7, No. 9, September 2006, pp. 671–681.

Bennett, Alex S., Luther Elliott, and Andrew Golub, "Opioid and Other Substance Misuse, Overdose Risk, and the Potential for Prevention Among a Sample of OEF/OIF Veterans in New York City," *Substance Use and Misuse*, Vol. 48, No. 10, July 2013, pp. 894–907.

Blanchard, Janice, Sarah B. Hunter, Karen Chan Osilla, Warren Stewart, Jennifer Walters, and Rosalie Liccardo Pacula, "A Systematic Review of the Prevention and Treatment of Prescription Drug Misuse," *Military Medicine*, Vol. 181, No. 5, May 2016, pp. 410–423.

Blondell, Richard D., Lisham Ashrafioun, Christina M. Dambra, Elisa M. Foschio, Amy L. Zielinski, and Daniel M. Salcedo, "A Clinical Trial Comparing Tapering Doses of Buprenorphine with Steady Doses for Chronic Pain and Co-Existent Opioid Addiction," *Journal of Addiction Medicine*, Vol. 4, No. 3, September 2010, pp. 140–146.

Bohnert, Amy S. B., Kathryn Roeder, and Mark A. Ilgen, "Unintentional Overdose and Suicide Among Substance Users: A Review of Overlap and Risk Factors," *Drug and Alcohol Dependence*, Vol. 110, No. 3, August 1, 2010, pp. 183–192.

Bray, Robert M., Kristine Rae Olmsted, and Jason William, "Misuse of Prescription Pain Medications in U.S. Active Duty Service Members," in Brenda K. Wiederhold, ed., *Wounds of War: Pain Syndromes—from Recruitment to Returning Troops*, Amsterdam: IOS Press, 2012, pp. 3–16.

Bray, Robert M., Michael R. Pemberton, Laurel L. Hourani, Michael Witt, Kristine L. Rae Olmsted, Janice M. Brown, BeLinda Weimer, Marian E. Lane, Mary Ellen Marsden, Scott Scheffler, Russ Vandermass-Peeler, Kimberly R. Aspinwall, Erin Anderson, Kathryn Spagnola, Kelly Close, Jennifer L. Gratton, Sara Calvin, and Michael Bradshaw, *2008 Department of Defense Survey of Health Related Behaviors Among Active Duty Military Personnel: A Component of the Defense Lifestyle Assessment Program (DLAP)*, September 2009. As of April 8, 2015: http://www.tricare.mil/tma/2008HealthBehaviors.pdf

Bray, Robert M., Michael R. Pemberton, Marian E. Lane, Laurel L. Hourani, Mark J. Mattiko, and Lorraine A. Babeu, "Substance Use and Mental Health Trends Among U.S. Military Active Duty Personnel: Key Findings from the 2008 DoD Health Behavior Survey," *Military Medicine*, Vol. 175, No. 6, June 2010, pp. 390–399. As of April 29, 2015: http://www.dtic.mil/cgi-bin/GetTRDoc?AD=ADA523045

Briggs, Andrew H., Karl Claxton, and Mark J. Sculpher, *Decision Modelling for Health Economic Evaluation*, Oxford, UK: Oxford University Press, 2006.

Buelow, A. K., R. Haggard, and R. J. Gatchel, "Additional Validation of the Pain Medication Questionnaire in a Heterogeneous Sample of Chronic Pain Patients," *Pain Practice*, Vol. 9, No. 6, November–December 2009, pp. 428–434.

Butler, Stephen F., Simon H. Budman, Kathrine C. Fernandez, Gilbert J. Fanciullo, and Robert N. Jamison, "Cross-Validation of a Screener to Predict Opioid Misuse in Chronic Pain Patients (SOAPP-R)," *Journal of Addiction Medicine*, Vol. 3, No. 2, June 1, 2009, pp. 66–73.

Butler, Stephen F., Simon H. Budman, Kathrine C. Fernandez, Brian Houle, Christine Benoit, Nathaniel Katz, and Robert N. Jamison, "Development and Validation of the Current Opioid Misuse Measure," *Pain*, Vol. 130, No. 1–2, July 2007, pp. 144–156.

Cantrill, Stephen V., Michael D. Brown, Russell J. Carlisle, Kathleen A. Delaney, Daniel P. Hays, Lewis S. Nelson, Robert E. O'Connor, AnnMarie Papa, Karl A. Sporer, Knox H. Todd, and Rhonda R. Whitson, "Clinical Policy: Critical Issues in the Prescribing of Opioids for Adult Patients in the Emergency Department," *Annals of Emergency Medicine*, Vol. 60, No. 4, October 2012, pp. 499–525. As of February 25, 2016:
http://www.acep.org/workarea/DownloadAsset.aspx?id=88197

Carlucci, Frank C., Deputy Secretary of Defense, memorandum 62884, December 28, 1981.

Chapman, C. Richard, David L. Lipschitz, Martin S. Angst, Roger Chou, Richard C. Denisco, Gary W. Donaldson, Perry G. Fine, Kathleen M. Foley, Rollin M. Gallagher, Aaron M. Gilson, J. David Haddox, Susan D. Horn, Charles E. Inturrisi, Susan S. Jick, Arthur G. Lipman, John D. Loeser, Meredith Noble, Linda Porter, Michael C. Rowbotham, Karen M. Schoelles, Dennis C. Turk, Ernest Volinn, Michael R. Von Korff, Lynn R. Webster, and Constance M. Weisner, "Opioid Pharmacotherapy for Chronic Non-Cancer Pain in the United States: A Research Guideline for Developing an Evidence-Base," *Journal of Pain*, Vol. 11, No. 9, September 2010, pp. 807–829.

Chief of Staff, Bureau of Medicine and Surgery, Department of the Navy, *Headquarters, Bureau of Medicine and Surgery Alcohol and Drug Prevention Program*, Bureau of Medicine and Surgery Instruction 5350.5, November 29, 2011. As of February 27, 2016:
http://www.med.navy.mil/directives/Internal%20Directives/5350.5.pdf

Chou, Roger, Gilbert J. Fanciullo, Perry G. Fine, Jeremy A. Adler, Jane C. Ballantyne, Pamela Davies, Marilee I. Donovan, David A. Fishbain, Kathy M. Foley, Jeffrey Fudin, Aaron M. Gilson, Alexander Kelter, Alexander Mauskop, Patrick G. O'Connor, Steven D. Passik, Gavril W. Pasternak, Russell K. Portenoy, Ben A. Rich, Richard G. Roberts, Knox H. Todd, and Christine Miaskowski, "Clinical Guidelines for the Use of Chronic Opioid Therapy in Chronic Noncancer Pain," *Journal of Pain*, Vol. 10, No. 2, February 2009, pp. 113–130.

Chou, Roger, Amir Qaseem, Vincenza Snow, Donald Casey, J. Thomas Cross, Jr., Paul Shekelle, and Douglas K. Owens, "Diagnosis and Treatment of Low Back Pain: A Joint Clinical Practice Guideline from the American College of Physicians and the American Pain Society," *Annals of Internal Medicine*, Vol. 147, 2007, pp. 478–491. As of February 28, 2016:
http://www.healthquality.va.gov/guidelines/Pain/lbp/

Cochran, G., B. Woo, W. H. Lo-Ciganic, A. J. Gordon, J. M. Donohue, and W. F. Gellad, "Defining Nonmedical Use of Prescription Opioids Within Health Care Claims: A Systematic Review," *Substance Abuse*, Vol. 36, No. 2, 2015, pp. 192–202.

Cucciare, Michael A., and Christine Timko, "Bridging the Gap Between Medical Settings and Specialty Addiction Treatment," *Addiction*, Vol. 110, No. 9, September 2015, pp. 1417–1419.

Deitz, D. K., R. F. Cook, and A. Hendrickson, "Preventing Prescription Drug Misuse: Field Test of the SmartRx Web Program," *Substance Use and Misuse*, Vol. 46, No. 5, 2011, pp. 678–686.

Deputy Commandant for Manpower and Reserve Affairs, Headquarters, U.S. Marine Corps, Department of the Navy, *Marine Corps Substance Abuse Program*, Marine Corps Order 5300.17, April 11, 2011. As of February 27, 2016:
http://www.med.navy.mil/sites/nmcphc/Documents/policy-and-instruction/mco-530017.pdf

Deputy Surgeon General of the Air Force, *Alcohol and Drug Abuse Prevention and Treatment (ADAPT) Program*, Air Force Instruction 44-121, April 11, 2011.

Director, Personal Readiness and Community Support Branch, Office of the Chief of Naval Operations, Department of the Navy, *Navy Alcohol and Drug Abuse Prevention and Control*, Chief of Naval Operations Instruction 5350.4D, June 4, 2009. As of February 27, 2016:
http://www.monterey.army.mil/Substance_Abuse/inc/navy.pdf

Dunn, Kate M., Kathleen W. Saunders, Carolyn M. Rutter, Caleb J. Banta-Green, Joseph O. Merrill, Mark D. Sullivan, Constance M. Weisner, Michael J. Silverberg, Cynthia I. Campbell, Bruce M. Psaty, and Michael Von Korff, "Opioid Prescriptions for Chronic Pain and Overdose: A Cohort Study," *Annals of Internal Medicine*, Vol. 152, No. 2, January 19, 2010, pp. 85–92.

Everingham, Susan S., and C. Peter Rydell, *Modeling the Demand for Cocaine*, Santa Monica, Calif.: RAND Corporation, MR-332-ONDCP/A/DPRC, 1994. As of February 25, 2016:
http://www.rand.org/pubs/monograph_reports/MR332.html

Fishbain, David A., Brandly Cole, John Lewis, Hubert L. Rosomoff, and R. Steele Rosomoff, "What Percentage of Chronic Nonmalignant Pain Patients Exposed to Chronic Opioid Analgesic Therapy Develop Abuse/Addiction and/or Aberrant Drug-Related Behaviors? A Structured Evidence-Based Review," *Pain Medicine*, Vol. 9, No. 4, May–June 2008, pp. 444–459.

Ghitza, U. E., and B. Tai, "Challenges and Opportunities for Integrating Preventive Substance-Use-Care Services in Primary Care Through the Affordable Care Act," *Journal of Health Care for the Poor and Underserved*, Vol. 25, No. 1 Suppl., February 2014, pp. 36–45.

Golub, Andrew, and Alex S. Bennett, "Prescription Opioid Initiation, Correlates, and Consequences Among a Sample of OEF/OIF Military Personnel," *Substance Use and Misuse*, Vol. 48, No. 10, July 2013, pp. 811–820.

Headquarters, Department of the Army, *Army 2020: Generating Health and Discipline in the Force Ahead of the Strategic Reset*, 2012a. As of February 25, 2016: http://www.army.mil/e2/c/downloads/235822.pdf

———, *The Army Substance Abuse Program*, Army Regulation 600-85, December 28, 2012b. As of February 26, 2016: http://www.apd.army.mil/pdffiles/r600_85.pdf

Hoare, Alexander, David G. Regan, and David P. Wilson, "Sampling and Sensitivity Analyses Tools (SaSAT) for Computational Modelling," *Theoretical Biology and Medical Modelling*, Vol. 5, No. 4, 2008.

Humphreys, Keith, and Richard G. Frank, "The Affordable Care Act Will Revolutionize Care for Substance Use Disorders in the United States," *Addiction*, Vol. 109, No. 12, December 2014, pp. 1957–1958.

Hutchinson, E., M. Catlin, C. H. Andrilla, L. M. Baldwin, and R. A. Rosenblatt, "Barriers to Primary Care Physicians Prescribing Buprenorphine," *Annals of Family Medicine*, Vol. 12, No. 2, March–April 2014, pp. 128–133.

Ilgen, Mark A., Kathryn M. Roeder, Linda Webster, Orion P. Mowbray, Brian E. Perron, Stephen T. Chermack, and Amy S. B. Bohnert, "Measuring Pain Medication Expectancies in Adults Treated for Substance Use Disorders," *Drug and Alcohol Dependence*, Vol. 115, No. 1–2, May 1, 2011, pp. 51–56.

Institute of Medicine, *Substance Use Disorders in the U.S. Armed Forces*, Washington, D.C.: National Academies Press, September 17, 2012. As of February 25, 2016: http://iom.nationalacademies.org/Reports/2012/ Substance-Use-Disorders-in-the-US-Armed-Forces.aspx

IOM—*See* Institute of Medicine.

Jeffery, D. D., *DEA Schedule II–IV Prescriptions Received by U.S. Active Duty Military Personnel in 2010*, American Society of Addiction Medicine's 43rd Annual Medical-Scientific Conference, April 2012.

Jeffery, D. D., L. A. Babeu, L. E. Nelson, M. Kloc, and K. Klette, "Prescription Drug Misuse Among U.S. Active Duty Military Personnel: A Secondary Analysis of the 2008 DoD Survey of Health Related Behaviors," *Military Medicine*, Vol. 178, No. 2, February 2013, pp. 180–195.

Jeffery, D. D., L. May, B. Luckey, B. M. Balison, and K. L. Klette, "Use and Abuse of Prescribed Opioids, Central Nervous System Depressants, and Stimulants Among U.S. Active Duty Military Personnel in FY 2010," *Military Medicine*, Vol. 179, No. 10, October 2014, pp. 1141–1148.

Knisely, Janet S., Martha J. Wunsch, Karen L. Cropsey, and Eleanor D. Campbell, "Prescription Opioid Misuse Index: A Brief Questionnaire to Assess Misuse," *Journal of Substance Abuse Treatment*, Vol. 35, No. 4, December 2008, pp. 380–386.

Levy, D. T., P. L. Mabry, Y. C. Wang, S. Gortmaker, T. T. Huang, T. Marsh, M. Moodie, and B. Swinburn, "Simulation Models of Obesity: A Review of the Literature and Implications for Research and Policy," *Obesity Reviews*, Vol. 12, No. 5, May 2011, pp. 378–394.

Looby, Alison, and Mitch Earleywine, "Psychometric Evaluation of a Prescription Stimulant Expectancy Questionnaire," *Experimental and Clinical Psychopharmacology*, Vol. 18, No. 4, August 2010, pp. 375–383.

Management of Opioid Therapy for Chronic Pain Working Group, *VA/DoD Clinical Practice Guideline for the Management of Opioid Therapy for Chronic Pain*, May 2010. As of February 25, 2016:
http://www.healthquality.va.gov/guidelines/Pain/cot/

Management of Substance Use Disorders Work Group, *VA/DoD Clinical Practice Guideline for Management of Substance Use Disorders*, August 2009.

Manchikanti, L., S. Abdi, S. Atluri, C. C. Balog, R. M. Benyamin, M. V. Boswell, K. R. Brown, B. M. Bruel, D. A. Bryce, P. A. Burks, A. W. Burton, A. K. Calodney, D. L. Caraway, K. A. Cash, P. J. Christo, K. S. Damron, S. Datta, T. R. Deer, S. Diwan, I. Eriator, F. J. Falco, B. Fellows, S. Geffert, C. G. Gharibo, S. E. Glaser, J. S. Grider, H. Hameed, M. Hameed, H. Hansen, M. E. Harned, S. M. Hayek, S. Helm II, J. A. Hirsch, J. W. Janata, A. D. Kaye, A. M. Kaye, D. S. Kloth, D. Koyyalagunta, M. Lee, Y. Malla, K. N. Manchikanti, C. D. McManus, V. Pampati, A. T. Parr, R. Pasupuleti, V. B. Patel, N. Sehgal, S. M. Silverman, V. Singh, H. S. Smith, L. T. Snook, D. R. Solanki, D. H. Tracy, R. Vallejo, and B. W. Wargo, "American Society of Interventional Pain Physicians (ASIPP) Guidelines for Responsible Opioid Prescribing in Chronic Non-Cancer Pain: Part I—Evidence Assessment," *Pain Physician*, Vol. 15, No. 3, Supp., July 2012a, pp. S1–S65.

———, "American Society of Interventional Pain Physicians (ASIPP) Guidelines for Responsible Opioid Prescribing in Chronic Non-Cancer Pain: Part 2—Guidance," *Pain Physician*, Vol. 15, No. 3, Supp., July 2012b, pp. S67–S116.

Martell, Bridget A., Patrick G. O'Connor, Robert D. Kerns, William C. Becker, Knashawn H. Morales, Thomas R. Kosten, and David A. Fiellin, "Systematic Review: Opioid Treatment for Chronic Back Pain—Prevalence, Efficacy, and Association with Addiction," *Annals of Internal Medicine*, Vol. 146, No. 2, January 16, 2007, pp. 116–127.

McLellan, A. Thomas, and Barbara J. Turner, "Chronic Noncancer Pain Management and Opioid Overdose: Time to Change Prescribing Practices," *Annals of Internal Medicine*, Vol. 152, January 19, 2010, pp. 123–124.

Moher, David, Alessandro Liberati, Jennifer Tetzlaff, Douglas G. Altman, and PRISMA Group, "Preferred Reporting Items for Systematic Reviews and Meta-Analyses: The PRISMA Statement," *Annals of Internal Medicine*, Vol. 151, No. 4, August 18, 2009, pp. 264–269.

Molfenter, Todd, Victor A. Capoccia, Michael G. Boyle, and Carol K. Sherbeck, "The Readiness of Addiction Treatment Agencies for Health Care Reform," *Substance Abuse Treatment, Prevention, and Policy*, Vol. 7, No. 16, 2012.

Morasco, B. J., S. Gritzner, L. Lewis, R. Oldham, D. C. Turk, and S. K. Dobscha, "Systematic Review of Prevalence, Correlates, and Treatment Outcomes for Chronic Non-Cancer Pain in Patients with Comorbid Substance Use Disorder," *Pain*, Vol. 152, No. 3, March 2011, pp. 488–497.

Nathan, M. L., "The Patient-Centered Medical Home in the Transformation from Healthcare to Health," *Military Medicine*, Vol. 178, No. 2, February 2013, pp. 126–127.

National Institute on Drug Abuse, *Principles of Drug Addiction Treatment: A Research-Based Guide*, 3rd ed., National Institutes of Health Publication 12-4180, 2012. As of February 25, 2016:
https://www.drugabuse.gov/publications/
principles-drug-addiction-treatment-research-based-guide-third-edition/
acknowledgments

Noble, Meredith, Stephen J. Tregear, Jonathan R. Treadwell, and Karen M. Schoelles, "Long-Term Opioid Therapy for Chronic Noncancer Pain: A Systematic Review and Meta-Analysis of Efficacy and Safety," *Journal of Pain and Symptom Management*, Vol. 35, No. 2, February 2008, pp. 214–228.

Nuckols, Teryl K., Laura Anderson, Ioana Popescu, Allison L. Diamant, Brian Doyle, Paul Di Capua, and Roger Chou, "Opioid Prescribing: A Systematic Review and Critical Appraisal of Guidelines for Chronic Pain," *Annals of Internal Medicine*, Vol. 160, No. 1, January 2014, pp. 38–47.

Office of the Army Surgeon General, *Pain Management Task Force Final Report: Providing a Standardized DoD and VHA Vision and Approach to Pain Management to Optimize the Care for Warriors and Their Families*, May 2010.

———, "ALARACT Changes to Length of Authorized Duration of Controlled Substance Prescriptions in MEDCOM Regulation 40-51," All Army Activities 062/2011, February 2011. As of September 6, 2016: https://www.garrison.hawaii.army.mil/asap/resources/Changes%20to%20 Length%20of%20Authorized%20Duration%20of%20Controlled%20 Substance%20Prescription_ALARACT_062_2011_.pdf

Office of the Assistant Secretary of Defense for Health Affairs, TRICARE Management Activity, "Protocol Approval," memorandum for CAPT Kevin Klette, Office of the Under Secretary of Defense for Personnel and Readiness, c. 2013.

Okie, Susan, "A Flood of Opioids, a Rising Tide of Deaths," *New England Journal of Medicine*, Vol. 363, No. 21, November 18, 2010, pp. 1981–1985.

Paddock, Susan M., Beau Kilmer, Jonathan P. Caulkins, Marika J. Booth, and Rosalie L. Pacula, "An Epidemiological Model for Examining Marijuana Use over the Life Course," *Epidemiology Research International*, Vol. 2012, January 2012, art. 520894.

Paulozzi, Leonard J., Christopher M. Jones, Karin A. Mack, and Rose A. Rudd, "Vital Signs: Overdoses of Prescription Opioid Pain Relievers—United States, 1999–2008," *Morbidity and Mortality Weekly Report*, Vol. 60, No. 43, November 4, 2011, pp. 1487–1492. As of February 25, 2016: http://www.cdc.gov/mmwr/preview/mmwrhtml/mm6043a4.htm

Paulozzi, Leonard J., Edwin M. Kilbourne, Nina G. Shah, Kurt B. Nolte, Hema A. Desai, Michael G. Landen, William Harvey, and Larry D. Loring, "A History of Being Prescribed Controlled Substances and Risk of Drug Overdose Death," *Pain Medicine*, Vol. 13, No. 1, January 2012, pp. 87–95.

Potter, J. S., A. Chakrabarti, C. P. Domier, M. P. Hillhouse, R. D. Weiss, and W. Ling, "Pain and Continued Opioid Use in Individuals Receiving Buprenorphine-Naloxone for Opioid Detoxification: Secondary Analyses from the Clinical Trials Network," *Journal of Substance Abuse Treatment*, Vol. 38, Supp. 1, June 2010, pp. S80–S86.

Prescription Drug Abuse Subcommittee, Behavioral Health Coordinating Committee, U.S. Department of Health and Human Services, *Addressing Prescription Drug Abuse in the United States: Current Activities and Future Opportunities*," c. September 2013. As of February 25, 2016: http://www.cdc.gov/drugoverdose/pdf/ hhs_prescription_drug_abuse_report_09.2013.pdf

Public Law 111-148, Patient Protection and Affordable Care Act, March 23, 2010. As of February 26, 2016: https://www.gpo.gov/fdsys/granule/PLAW-111publ148/PLAW-111publ148/ content-detail.html

Rapp, Richard C., Amy L. Otto, D. Timothy Lane, Cristina Redko, Sue McGatha, and Robert G. Carlson, "Improving Linkage with Substance Abuse Treatment Using Brief Case Management and Motivational Interviewing," *Drug and Alcohol Dependence*, Vol. 94, No. 1–3, April 1, 2008, pp. 172–182.

Rawson, R. A., P. Marinelli-Casey, M. D. Anglin, A. Dickow, Y. Frazier, C. Gallagher, G. P. Galloway, J. Herrell, A. Huber, M. J. McCann, J. Obert, S. Pennell, C. Reiber, D. Vandersloot, and J. Zweben, "A Multi-Site Comparison of Psychosocial Approaches for the Treatment of Methamphetamine Dependence," *Addiction*, Vol. 99, No. 6, June 2004, pp. 708–717.

Rawson, R. A., S. J. Shoptaw, J. L. Obert, M. J. McCann, A. L. Hasson, P. J. Marinelli-Casey, P. R. Brethen, and W. Ling, "An Intensive Outpatient Approach for Cocaine Abuse Treatment: The Matrix Model," *Journal of Substance Abuse Treatment*, Vol. 12, No. 2, March–April 1995, pp. 117–127.

Reifler, Liza M., Danna Droz, J. Elise Bailey, Sidney H. Schnoll, Reginald Fant, Richard C. Dart, and Becki Bucher Bartelson, "Do Prescription Monitoring Programs Impact State Trends in Opioid Abuse/Misuse?" *Pain Medicine*, Vol. 13, No. 3, March 2012, pp. 434–442.

Rossi, C., "The Role of Dynamic Modeling in Drug Abuse Epidemiology," *Bulletin on Narcotics*, Vol. LIV, No. 1–2, 2002, pp. 33–44.

Rutter, C. M., A. M. Zaslavsky, and E. J. Feuer, "Dynamic Microsimulation Models for Health Outcomes: A Review," *Medical Decision Making*, Vol. 31, No. 1, January–February 2011, pp. 10–18.

Rydell, C. Peter, Jonathan P. Caulkins, and Susan S. Everingham, "Enforcement or Treatment? Modeling the Relative Efficacy of Alternatives for Controlling Cocaine," *Operations Research*, Vol. 44, No. 5, September–October 1996, pp. 687–695.

Rydell, C. Peter, and Susan S. Everingham, *Controlling Cocaine: Supply Versus Demand Programs*, Santa Monica, Calif.: RAND Corporation, MR-331-ONDCP/A/DPRC, 1994. As of February 25, 2016: http://www.rand.org/pubs/monograph_reports/MR331.html

SAMHSA—*See* Substance Abuse and Mental Health Services Administration.

Seal, Karen H., Ying Shi, Gregory Cohen, Beth E. Cohen, Shira Maguen, Erin E. Krebs, and Thomas C. Neylan, "Association of Mental Health Disorders with Prescription Opioids and High-Risk Opioid Use in US Veterans of Iraq and Afghanistan," *JAMA*, Vol. 307, No. 9, March 7, 2012, pp. 940–947.

Secretary of the Army, *The Army Substance Abuse Program*, Army Regulation 600-85, February 2, 2009.

Servies, Tammy, Zheng Hu, Angelia Eick-Cost, and Jean Lin Otto, "Substance Use Disorders in the U.S. Armed Forces, 2000–2011," *Medical Surveillance Monthly Report*, Vol. 19, No. 11, November 2012, pp. 11–16.

Shallenberger, F., "Selective Compartmental Dominance: An Explanation for a Noninfectious, Multifactorial Etiology for Acquired Immune Deficiency Syndrome (AIDS), and a Rationale for Ozone Therapy and Other Immune Modulating Therapies," *Medical Hypotheses*, Vol. 50, No. 1, January 1998, pp. 67–80.

Sigmon, S. C., K. E. Dunn, G. J. Badger, S. H. Heil, and S. T. Higgins, "Brief Buprenorphine Detoxification for the Treatment of Prescription Opioid Dependence: A Pilot Study," *Addictive Behaviors*, Vol. 34, No. 3, March 2009, pp. 304–311.

Smith, M. Y., W. Irish, J. Wang, J. D. Haddox, and R. C. Dart, "Detecting Signals of Opioid Analgesic Abuse: Application of a Spatial Mixed Effect Poisson Regression Model Using Data from a Network of Poison Control Centers," *Pharmacoepidemiology and Drug Safety*, Vol. 17, No. 11, November 2008, pp. 1050–1059.

Smith, Richard C., Cathy Frank, Joseph C. Gardiner, Lois Lamerato, and Kathryn M. Rost, "Pilot Study of a Preliminary Criterion Standard for Prescription Opioid Misuse," *American Journal on Addictions*, Vol. 19, No. 6, November–December 2010, pp. 523–528.

Sonnenberg, F. A., and J. R. Beck, "Markov Models in Medical Decision Making: A Practical Guide," *Medical Decision Making*, Vol. 13, No. 4, October–December 1993, pp. 322–338.

Starrels, Joanna L., William C. Becker, Daniel P. Alford, Alok Kapoor, Arthur Robinson Williams, and Barbara J. Turner, "Systematic Review: Treatment Agreements and Urine Drug Testing to Reduce Opioid Misuse in Patients with Chronic Pain," *Annals of Internal Medicine*, Vol. 152, No. 11, June 1, 2010, pp. 712–720.

Substance Abuse and Mental Health Services Administration, Office of Applied Studies, *Results from the 2001 National Household Survey on Drug Abuse*, Rockville, Md., SMA02-3758, 2002. As of February 25, 2016: http://homeless.samhsa.gov/resource/results-from-the-2001-national-household-survey-on-drug-abuse-volume-i-summary-of-national-findings-volume-ii-technical-appendices-and-selected-data-tables-21735.aspx

———, Center for Substance Abuse Treatment, *Clinical Guidelines for the Use of Buprenorphine in the Treatment of Opioid Addiction: A Treatment Improvement Protocol TIP 40*, Rockville, Md., SMA04-3939, September 2004. As of February 25, 2016: http://store.samhsa.gov/product/TIP-40-Clinical-Guidelines-for-the-Use-of-Buprenorphine-in-the-Treatment-of-Opioid-Addiction/SMA07-3939

———, Center for Substance Abuse Treatment, *Medication-Assisted Treatment for Opioid Addiction in Opioid Treatment Programs: A Treatment Improvement Protocol TIP 43*, Rockville, Md., SMA12-4214, November 2008. As of February 25, 2016: http://store.samhsa.gov/product/TIP-43-Medication-Assisted-Treatment-for-Opioid-Addiction-in-Opioid-Treatment-Programs/SMA12-4214

———, Center for Substance Abuse Treatment, *Treatment for Stimulant Use Disorders*, Rockville, Md., Treatment Improvement Protocol 33, SMA09-4209, June 2009. As of February 25, 2016: http://store.samhsa.gov/product/TIP-33-Treatment-for-Stimulant-Use-Disorder/SMA09-4209

———, Center for Behavioral Health Statistics and Quality, *Results from the 2010 National Survey on Drug Use and Health: Summary of National Findings*, Rockville, Md., SMA11-4658, 2011. As of February 25, 2016: http://www.samhsa.gov/data/sites/default/files/NSDUHNationalFindingsResults2010-web/2k10ResultsRev/NSDUHresultsRev2010.pdf

———, *Managing Chronic Pain in Adults in Recovery with or in Recovery from Substance Use Disorders: A Treatment Improvement Protocol*, Rockville, Md., Treatment Improvement Protocol 54, SMA12-4671, 2012. As of February 25, 2016: http://store.samhsa.gov/product/TIP-54-Managing-Chronic-Pain-in-Adults-With-or-in-Recovery-From-Substance-Use-Disorders/SMA13-4671

———, Center for Behavioral Health Statistics and Quality, *Results from the 2013 National Survey on Drug Use and Health: Summary of National Findings*, Rockville, Md., SMA14-4863, September 2014. As of February 25, 2016: http://store.samhsa.gov/product/Results-from-the-2013-National-Survey-on-Drug-Use-and-Health-Summary-of-National-Findings/SMA14-4863

———, *Clinical Use of Extended-Release Injectable Naltrexone in the Treatment of Opioid Use Disorder: A Brief Guide*, Rockville, Md., SMA14-4892R, January 2015. As of February 25, 2016: http://store.samhsa.gov/product/Clinical-Use-of-Extended-Release-Injectable-Naltrexone-in-the-Treatment-of-Opioid-Use-Disorder-A-Brief-Guide/SMA14-4892R

Thomas, Cindy Parks, Sharon Reif, Sayeda Haq, Stanley S. Wallack, Alexander Hoyt, and Grant A. Ritter, "Use of Buprenorphine for Addiction Treatment: Perspectives of Addiction Specialists and General Psychiatrists," *Psychiatric Services*, Vol. 59, No. 8, August 2008, pp. 909–916.

Thorson, D., P. Biewen, B. Bonte, H. Epstein, B. Haake, C. Hansen, M. Hooten, J. Hora, C. Johnson, F. Keeling, A. Kokayeff, E. Krebs, C. Myers, B. Nelson, M. P. Noonan, C. Reznikoff, M. Thiel, A. Trujillo, S. Van Pelt, and J. Wainio, "Acute Pain Assessment and Opioid Prescribing Protocol," *Health Care Protocol*, 2013.

Turk, D. C., K. S. Swanson, and R. J. Gatchel, "Predicting Opioid Misuse by Chronic Pain Patients: A Systematic Review and Literature Synthesis," *Clinical Journal of Pain*, Vol. 24, No. 6, July–August 2008, pp. 497–508.

Under Secretary of Defense for Personnel and Readiness, *Command Notification Requirements to Dispel Stigma in Providing Mental Health Care to Service Members*, Department of Defense Instruction 6490.08, August 17, 2011a. As of February 27, 2016:
http://www.dtic.mil/whs/directives/corres/pdf/649008p.pdf

———, *Deployment Health*, Department of Defense Instruction 6490.03, August 11, 2006, certified current as of September 30, 2011b. As of February 27, 2016:
http://www.dtic.mil/whs/directives/corres/pdf/649003p.pdf

———, *DoD Civilian Employee Drug-Free Workplace Program*, Department of Defense Instruction 1010.09, June 22, 2012a. As of February 27, 2016:
http://www.dtic.mil/whs/directives/corres/pdf/101009p.pdf

———, *Military Personnel Drug Abuse Testing Program (MPDATP)*, Department of Defense Instruction 1010.01, September 13, 2012b. As of February 27, 2016:
http://www.dtic.mil/whs/directives/corres/pdf/101001p.pdf

———, *Problematic Substance Use by DoD Personnel*, Department of Defense Instruction 1010.04, February 20, 2014. As of February 27, 2016:
http://www.dtic.mil/whs/directives/corres/pdf/101004p.pdf

U.S. Marine Corps, *Marine Corps Drug and Alcohol Abuse Prevention and Treatment Programs*, Navy Marine Corps 2931, undated. As of February 27, 2016:
http://www.marforres.marines.mil/Portals/116/Docs/MCCS/MFS/Docs/DDRSACO/NAVMC2931.pdf

Warner, Margaret, Li Hui Chen, Diane M. Makuc, Robert N. Anderson, and Arialdi M. Miniño, "Drug Poisoning Deaths in the United States, 1980–2008," National Center for Health Statistics Data Brief 81, December 2011. As of February 25, 2016:
http://www.cdc.gov/nchs/data/databriefs/db81.htm

Webster, L. R., and R. M. Webster, "Predicting Aberrant Behaviors in Opioid-Treated Patients: Preliminary Validation of the Opioid Risk Tool," *Pain Medicine*, Vol. 6, No. 6, November–December 2005, pp. 432–442.

Weinstein, M. C., B. O'Brien, J. Hornberger, J. Jackson, M. Johannesson, C. McCabe, and B. R. Luce, "Principles of Good Practice for Decision Analytic Modeling in Health-Care Evaluation: Report of the ISPOR Task Force on Good Research Practices—Modeling Studies," *Value in Health*, Vol. 6, No. 1, January–February 2003, pp. 9–17.

Weinstein, Milton C., Edmond L. Toy, Eileen A. Sandberg, Peter J. Neumann, John S. Evans, Karen M. Kuntz, John D. Graham, and James K. Hammitt, "Modeling for Health Care and Other Policy Decisions: Uses, Roles, and Validity," *Value in Health*, Vol. 4, No. 5, September–October 2001, pp. 348–361.

Weiss, Roger D., Jennifer Sharpe Potter, David A. Fiellin, Marilyn Byrne, Hilary S. Connery, William Dickinson, John Gardin, Margaret L. Griffin, Marc N. Gourevitch, Deborah L. Haller, Albert L. Hasson, Zhen Huang, Petra Jacobs, Andrzej S. Kosinski, Robert Lindblad, Elinore F. McCance-Katz, Scott E. Provost, Jeffrey Selzer, Eugene C. Somoza, Susan C. Sonne, and Walter Ling, "Adjunctive Counseling During Brief and Extended Buprenorphine-Naloxone Treatment for Prescription Opioid Dependence: A 2-Phase Randomized Controlled Trial," *Archives of General Psychiatry*, Vol. 68, No. 12, December 2011, pp. 1238–1246.

Wu, P. C., C. Lang, N. K. Hasson, S. H. Linder, and D. J. Clark, "Opioid Use in Young Veterans," *Journal of Opioid Management*, Vol. 6, No. 2, March–April 2010, pp. 133–139.